REMEDIAL YOGA

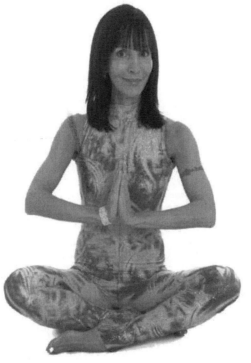

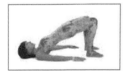 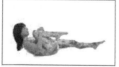 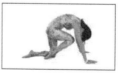 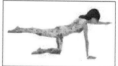

A fully illustrated breakdown of seventy yoga poses, with medically beneficial, rewarding and effective results.
A safe and practical yoga programme, designed with you in mind, brought to you by the author of
"Rosie's Armchair Exercises"

ROSITA EVANS

To order additional copies of this book, contact:
Xlibris LLC
0-800-056-3182
www.xlibrispublishing.co.uk
Orders@ Xlibrispublishing.co.uk
307231

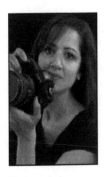

Photography by
Harpreet Castleton of
Magenta Photography.com

Foreword
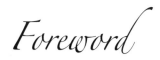

"Rosie's Remedial Yoga" is an excellent insight into how Yoga should be performed, effectively and safely.

Sadly, as we get older our joints normally become stiffer, and as such they become more vulnerable to aches and pains. The practice of Yoga can slow down this stiffness, and hence potential aches and pains, if done on a consistent basis. Because Yoga has also been in existence and arguably practiced for thousands of years, the long term benefits have been well documented, not only in regard to the physical side, but also the mental and emotional side.

I have personally known Rosie for many years, and she is truly professional and an expert in her field. She has managed to create a yoga programme with safety as the main focus, and that is what makes this book unique.

Her passion and experience is seen by many of my patients, all of whom have nothing but praise for her. If you embrace this book and consistently work on her exercises, I have no doubt that it will help your flexibility, muscle strength and state of mind.

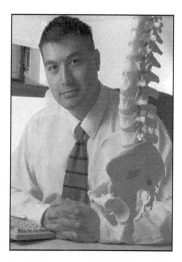

Dr Solomon Abrahams, PhD, MSc, BSc, MCSP, SRP
Consultant Physiotherapist

About the Author

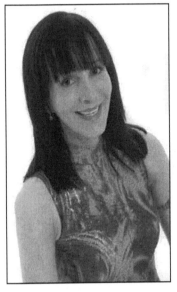

Rosie qualified as a Fitness Instructor and Personal Trainer in 1986, and went on to specialise in Hatha Yoga, which has been a passion of hers since childhood.

She is interested in all aspects of health and fitness, including complementary and holistic therapies. She has a particular interest in remedial yoga, and has studied and researched this subject for many years. The safety of her students is of paramount importance to Rosie, and she has therefore removed all potentially dangerous postures from her classes, and from this book.

She has also spent some time working with a large physiotherapy and sports injury practice, teaching remedial yoga to patients as part of their recovery programme.

She is "Fitness Expert" for Woman's Weekly magazine, one of the best selling weekly women's magazines in the United Kingdom, and has also written health-related articles for the Diabetes Research Foundation.

Born in London, Rosie now lives in Harrow, Middlesex, in the United Kingdom. She is the principal Yoga instructor for two large gyms in Harrow, and has been teaching yoga for more than 20 years.

Already a published author, her first book entitled "Rosie's Armchair Exercises" was published in 2002.

Contents

Disclaimer

Before you start this yoga programme:

- Always consult your GP before starting a new fitness programme if you do not exercise regularly.

- Do not attempt the exercises if you are recovering from an injury or illness, without first consulting your doctor.

- Always stop an exercise if it causes pain.

- Do not attempt these exercises if you have been drinking alcohol.

- Wait at least two hours after eating before attempting the exercises.

- Although many of the exercises are fine for use in pregnancy, this exercise programme has not been made with pregnancy in mind, so we cannot recommend that you follow them.

- Make sure you are warm and wearing loose, non-restrictive clothing.

- You will need a yoga mat or a non-slip exercise mat.

- **You are advised to read through the directions for each pose completely at least once before attempting it. Pay particular attention to the "Note" section at the end of each pose, where guidance and advice are given.**

A Brief Introduction to Yoga

Yoga originated thousands of years ago in India. The oldest archaeological evidence of its existence is provided by a number of stone figures in yogic postures, which were excavated from the Indus Valley and believed to date from around 3000BC.

Yoga was first brought to Europe in the 1800's by colonial administrators, soldiers and scholars returning from residence in India. This led to visits to Europe in the early 1900's by leading yogis from India, who toured and demonstrated yoga. Interest continued to grow, and in the 1980's it culminated in an explosion of yoga classes in the west, particularly Britain and the USA. It is currently considered the most popular form of exercise in the western world.

The underlying purpose of Yoga is to reunite our spiritual and mental self with our physical self, thereby making us "whole". The actual word YOGA means literally "joining".

Anyone can practice Yoga. You don't need special equipment or clothes – just a small amount of space and a strong desire for a healthier lifestyle, and a fitter body. The Yoga postures exercise every part of the body, stretching and toning the muscles and joints, the spine and the entire skeletal system. By releasing physical and mental tension, they also liberate vast resources of energy. The breathing exercises revitalise the body, leaving you feeling calm and refreshed.

In recent years, medical research has begun to pay attention to the beneficial effects of Yoga. Studies have shown, for example, that the relaxation poses can relieve high blood pressure, and that the regular practice of Yoga can help conditions such as arthritis, chronic fatigue, asthma, digestive problems and some heart conditions. One six-month study on the effects of Hatha Yoga demonstrated a significant increase in lung capacity and respiration, reduced bodyweight and measurements, and an improved ability to resist stress.

I have included in this book many poses with proven medical benefits – not only those I have just touched upon, but also poses to:

- strengthen the spinal muscles
- mobilise the hips
- help reduce the effects of Osteoporosis/loss of bone density
- improve posture
- stimulate the circulatory system reducing the risk of deep vein thrombosis and varicose veins
- help prevent incontinence and prolapse of the bladder or bowel.

Many people are first drawn to Yoga as a way to keep their bodies fit, strong and supple. The regular practice of Yoga will give your body not only flexibility, but a longer, leaner more streamlined look. Others come seeking help or relief for a specific complaint, like tension or backache. Whatever your reason, Yoga can work for you, on both a physical and a mental level.

There are four main physical benefits to regularly practising Hatha Yoga:

- It will strengthen, tone and stretch your muscles
- It will keep your joints strong and mobile
- It will improve your levels of flexibility and suppleness
- It will maintain a healthy circulation

Safety

Obviously, when yoga was first brought to the UK back in the 19th Century, we did not have the benefits of CT scans, X-Rays, or the vast array of medical technology and resources we now have at our fingertips. As a result, we were not aware at that time of just how easy it is to damage the human body. It is my personal belief that certain yoga postures practiced today can be potentially harmful and can cause injury. I believe that yoga should be allowed to "evolve" and develop in line with our ever-improving medical knowledge. I have therefore removed those postures that I feel could be dangerous from my yoga practice, in order to make this book as safe and enjoyable as possible. So, for example, I will not be asking you to stand on your head, or your shoulders, both of which can cause compression of the very delicate vertebrae of your neck. Other vulnerable areas of your body, like your spine and your wrists, will not be placed at risk by the poses in this book.

You may have heard or read about Salon Stroke Syndrome. This is where, by exerting stress on the neck – for instance at a hair salon where the neck is arched backward over a sink – can cause a kink or a tear in one of the main arteries of the neck, diminishing the blood supply to the brain, triggering a stroke. If the brain is deprived of its normal blood flow long enough, the damage can be permanent. Certain yoga poses require the same kind of head position, where the neck is arched back and the weight of the head is not supported. Therefore, I have removed, or modified, any pose that involves arching the neck backwards.

I advise you to read through the directions for each pose completely at least once before attempting it. Pay particular attention to the "Note" section at the end of each pose, where guidance and advice are given.

One more important point: Feel free to adapt or modify any of the poses in this book – if, by changing the pose slightly, you can make it more comfortable for yourself, then by all means do so. I believe yoga is a very individual art form, and we are all different, so what might work for one person may not work so well for another. Make this programme work for you.

Nothing is more important to me than your wellbeing and safety.

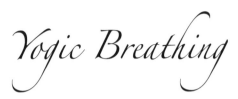

Yogic Breathing

Ideally, in Hatha Yoga you breathe through your nose. However, if you find this difficult – for example if you have an allergy or a cold, do not stress yourself out by trying to breathe through your nose. Do what feels most natural and comfortable for you – perhaps in through your nose and out through your mouth, or in and out through your mouth if you prefer. The most important aspect of your breathing is that you focus on filling your lungs completely on your breath in, and emptying your lungs completely on your breath out.

Generally, we are using just two-thirds of our lung capacity as we breathe. We try to correct this in our yoga practice so be constantly aware of your breathing, trying to slow it down, taking long full breaths in and out, using the whole of your lung capacity. Deep breathing in Yoga is important for many reasons:

- It improves mental control
- It deepens the beneficial effects of the postures
- It restores the natural balance of the body's energy flow
- It lowers the blood pressure
- It helps to lower stress levels and enables you to control stress more effectively
- It can help minimise conditions such as asthma and hypertension

But mainly:

- It stimulates self-healing and boosts the immune system. We are supposed to be a totally self-contained organism, and have within ourselves everything we need to heal us when we are ill. This self-healing process is at its strongest when we are sleeping and deeply relaxed (which is why, when we are unwell, we want to sleep).

Note: For the purposes of this book, where the term "deep breath" is written, it refers to a complete breath – i.e. both inhale AND exhale.

Relaxation

Life today is stressful for us all, and we can easily forget the art of relaxation, or simply not make time to relax. Stress, when left unchecked, can cause depression, physical illness, and can ultimately be a killer. While, of course, we can never totally eliminate stress from our lives, we **can** learn to control it, so that it doesn't take over our lives. The breathing and relaxation techniques used in Hatha Yoga can play a very large and important part in this process.

Hand Positions

Two hand positions will be used throughout this book: **Prayer Pose** and **Temple Pose.**

Prayer Pose:

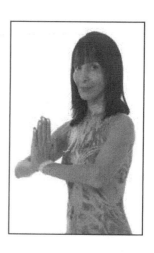

- The palms of your hands come together, fingertips facing the ceiling. Your thumbs should be at breastbone level, with your elbows out to each side and level with each other. Do not let your hands touch your body.

Temple Pose:

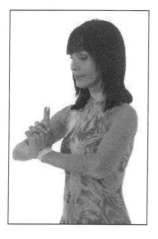

- This pose is used to help keep the hands together, in poses where **Prayer Pose** would be difficult to sustain. From **Prayer Pose**, simply link all your fingers together and curl them in, and cross your thumbs. Then extend just your index fingers, keeping them together and straight.

POSES

Suggested use of this book

- Always start your yoga workout with "Rejuvenator Stretch", which can be found in the Energising section. This stretch will warm your muscles and prepare you, both in mind and body, for your yoga practice.

- Always finish your yoga workout by either repeating "Rejuvenator Stretch", or "Corpse Pose", which can be found in the Relaxation section. This will allow your body to relax after your yoga practice, and give you time to return, both physically and spiritually, to your normal day routine.

- Use Child Pose, also in the Relaxation section, as often as you wish during your yoga practice to relax your body momentarily between poses.

- For a full yoga progamme, choose 2 poses from each section. Alternatively, tailor your yoga programme to suit your own needs.

- Yoga can be safely practiced on a daily basis. For the full effects, practice yoga at least 3 times a week for a minimum of 30 minutes.

SECTION 1

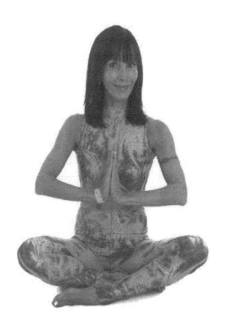

ENERGISING POSES

ENERGISING POSES

The primary function of energising poses is to stimulate the circulatory system. They will help to keep your circulation working efficiently, and ensure that your heart – which, after all, is a muscle – and your lungs, are doing their job as well as they should.

Energising poses are also great workouts for the main muscle groups of the body – strengthening and lengthening muscles, enabling them to work at their most optimum level. They are best done at the start of your yoga workout, as they will ensure your muscles are warm and stretched, and prepared for exercise.

Rejuvenator Stretch

Rejuvenator is essentially a "training pose", to ensure that you are taking deep, slow, full breaths in and out. The aim is to match your arm movements to your breathing, making both as slow as possible. For this reason, it is recommended that you start every yoga session with Rejuvenator, to make sure that your breathing is correct from the start.

Rejuvenator is also a wonderful stretch which can be done at any time – not just in your yoga routine. If done first thing in the morning, as soon as you get out of bed, it can help you focus and prepare for the day ahead. And done last thing at night, before you get into bed, it can help prepare your body for a good night's sleep.

- Stand tall, with your feet hip-width apart. Make sure you have an equal amount of bodyweight on each leg (it's very easy to sink onto one hip, without even realising you are doing it!) Keep your tailbone tucked under, so that you are not arching your back, draw your shoulders back and lengthen your neck.

- Breathe in, slowly raising both arms out to your sides and then up towards the ceiling as you do so. Reaching the top, link your fingers together and breathe out as you stretch both hands up to the ceiling. Then, take a deep breath in and stretch even higher. Finally breathe out as you bring your arms slowly back down to your sides.

- On your next breath in raise just your right arm, keeping it as straight as possible and reaching continually through to your fingertips. Breathe out and stretch your right arm and upper body over on to a diagonal – your fingers reaching for the top corner of the room. (You should feel the stretch running down your right-hand side). Breathe in as you return your body to an upright position, your fingertips reaching high for the ceiling, and then breathe out as you return your arm down to your side.

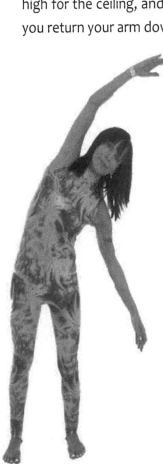

- Repeat with your left arm.

- Finally, to complete the pose, repeat once more with both arms.

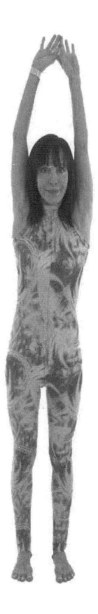

Note: Every arm movement in this pose is matched by your breathing. Your aim is to make your breathing as slow and as deep as possible, synchronising each movement with the breath. Check from time to time that you are not arching your back, by keeping your tailbone tucked under.

Chair Pose

Chair Pose *is wonderful for strengthening the thighs, while adding length to the muscle at the same time. Your thigh muscles will become longer, leaner and more powerful, and your knees will become stronger.*

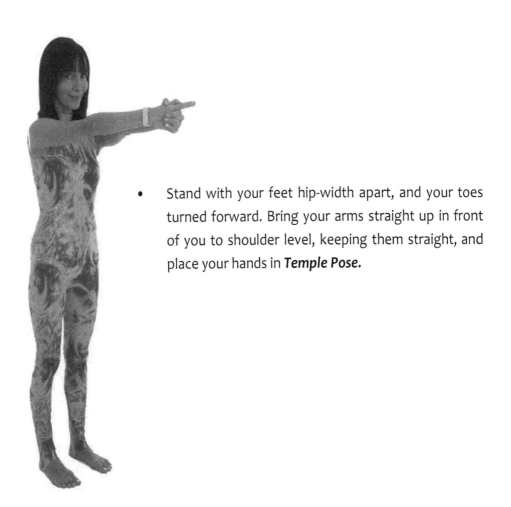

- Stand with your feet hip-width apart, and your toes turned forward. Bring your arms straight up in front of you to shoulder level, keeping them straight, and place your hands in **Temple Pose.**

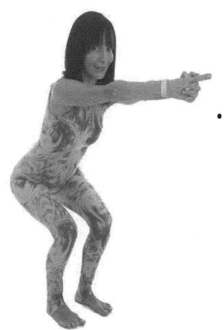

- Now, imagine a chair placed right behind you and slowly start to bend your knees, allowing your bottom to come out behind you as though you were going to sit on your imaginary chair. The lower you go the better, but never bring your bottom down lower than the level of your knees. Your upper body will come forward slightly.

- Keep your back straight throughout the pose, by drawing your shoulders back, and pressing your tailbone out behind you. Your arms remain straight out in front of you at shoulder level. Now, push your bodyweight back onto your heels – you should be able to "peel" your toes off the floor. (Try this for a few seconds, but make sure you then return your toes to the floor, keeping your weight over your heels).

- You are now in **Chair Pose**. Aim to hold this pose for at least 8-10 deep breaths, slowly increasing this number as you get stronger.

Note: Make sure your thighs and knees remain apart. Your knees must remain over your toes, and must not come together.

Mountain Pose

*This pose is deceptive! You may not feel like much is happening – but you are giving your heart and circulation a fantastic workout! It is also a wonderful pose to strengthen the muscles that surround and support the shoulders. **Mountain Pose** is performed in two stages – stay with the basic pose until you feel ready for the elevated version.*

Stage 1: Basic Mountain Pose

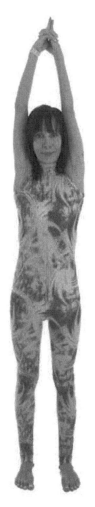

- Stand with your feet hip-width apart, toes turned forward. Take a deep breath in as you stretch both arms out to your sides and up towards the ceiling. Link your hands into **Temple Pose**, and as you breathe out stretch them as high as you can. Keep your arms either side of your ears throughout the pose.

- Make sure you do not arch your back – your tailbone should remain tucked under throughout this pose.

- Take 8-10 deep breaths, and then slowly return your arms to your sides and release the pose.

Note: Your arms will begin to feel 'heavy' – you might even feel "pins & needles", but this is entirely normal, and a sign that your circulation is working harder. Focus on your breathing to help you manage this.

Stage 2: Elevated Mountain Pose

*This part of the pose is optional, and can be added at the end of the basic pose if you wish to work harder! In addition to the benefits listed earlier, **Elevated Mountain** will strengthen the ankles and arches of your feet – a great pose if you do a lot of running or sports.*

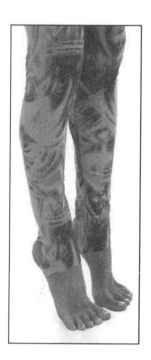

- Once you have completed your breaths in basic **Mountain Pose**, elevate the pose by lifting high onto your toes. Try not to roll out on your ankles – a good way of preventing this is by pushing your bodyweight onto your big toes.

- Hold your **Elevated Mountain Pose** for a further 5 deep breaths before slowly returning your arms to your sides, your heels to the floor and releasing the pose.

Note: If you are wobbling, try to fix your gaze on something not moving ahead of you – for instance a picture on a wall, or a piece of furniture – focussing on one still spot should help to keep you balanced.

Sumo Pose

Sumo is a strong pose and a great workout for the thighs, torso and shoulders in particular. It is quite a long and strenuous pose, requiring control and focus, but gives you fabulous results - especially if you wish to tighten your waist and firm up your thighs!

- Take your feet wide apart – at least one metre – and turn your toes slightly out. Now bend your knees and drop down about 8-10 inches. Keep your tailbone tucked under, shoulders back and knees turned out and over your toes throughout the whole pose. Bring your hands into **Prayer Pose** at chest level.

- Keeping your body upright, slide your bodyweight over to your right-hand side, allowing your left leg to straighten completely.

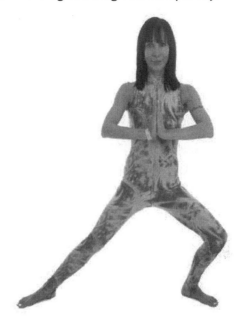

You should be aware of your bodyweight on your right thigh, strengthening and lengthening the muscles there. Hold for two deep breaths, and then slide directly over to your left-hand side, allowing your right leg to straighten completely. Again, hold for two deep breaths.

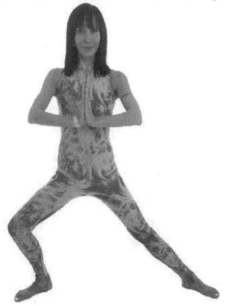

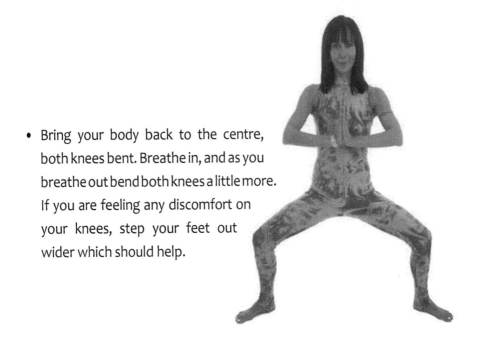

- Bring your body back to the centre, both knees bent. Breathe in, and as you breathe out bend both knees a little more. If you are feeling any discomfort on your knees, step your feet out wider which should help.

- Repeat the above stage, sliding your bodyweight to each side. Because you have now increased the bend in your knees, you will be aware of the extra workload placed on your thighs.

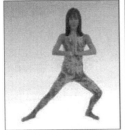 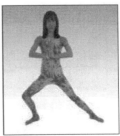

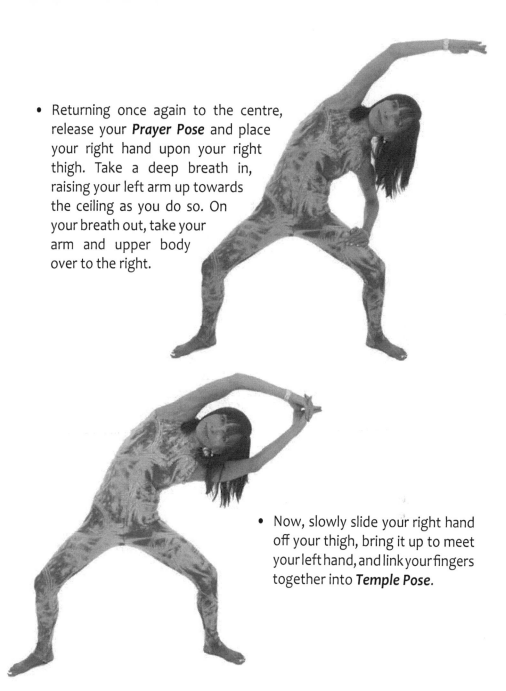

- Returning once again to the centre, release your **Prayer Pose** and place your right hand upon your right thigh. Take a deep breath in, raising your left arm up towards the ceiling as you do so. On your breath out, take your arm and upper body over to the right.

- Now, slowly slide your right hand off your thigh, bring it up to meet your left hand, and link your fingers together into **Temple Pose**.

- Keep your arms as straight as you can at this stage. You have now activated your intercostal muscles (situated between the ribs) and also the obliques (waist muscles). Try to stay in this position for 3 breaths before slowly returning your torso to its upright position. Make sure you do not allow your legs to straighten, or your upper body to turn down to face the floor. Draw back with your upper arm and shoulder continually to prevent this.

- Return your hands to *Prayer Pose*, and repeat the above stage, going to your left.

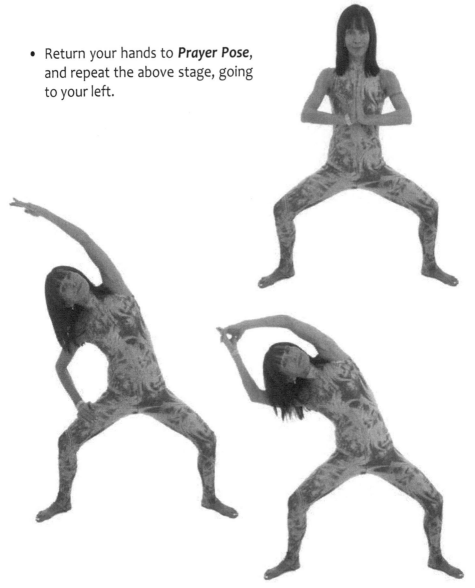

- Return to the centre, and place your hands in **Prayer Pose**. Take a deep breath in as you raise your **Prayer Pose** to the ceiling, and as you breathe out slowly release your arms back to your sides and straighten your legs.

Note: It is very important to keep both knees turned out, over your toes, throughout this pose. Take great care not to allow them to "roll in". If you find the latter stage – where you take your hand off your thigh - difficult, allow your bodyweight to remain supported by keeping your hand on your thigh. With practice you will soon find you can complete the pose unsupported.

Triangle Pose

Triangle is both energising and strengthening, focussing on the shoulders, spine, waist and hips. Triangle is all about straight body lines and stretching, and it will increase flexibility considerably. Reverse Triangle, which is linked to its sister pose – Triangle – introduces a gentle twist in the torso and will not only tighten up your waist but also strengthen the intercostal muscles, giving you a much smoother and tighter torso. By strengthening the intercostals, which are responsible for expanding and contracting the ribcage as you breathe, Reverse Triangle can also increase lung capacity.

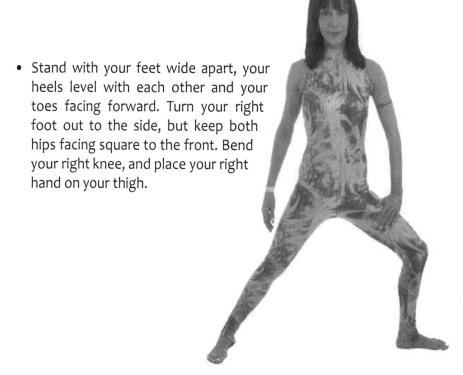

- Stand with your feet wide apart, your heels level with each other and your toes facing forward. Turn your right foot out to the side, but keep both hips facing square to the front. Bend your right knee, and place your right hand on your thigh.

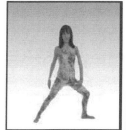 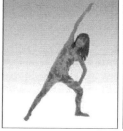 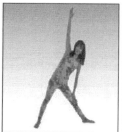 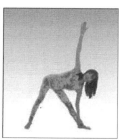

- Breathe in as you raise your left arm up, and breathe out as you stretch your arm over onto a diagonal – you are aiming to be in a straight diagonal line from your fingertips down to your left foot. Hold this position for two deep breaths.

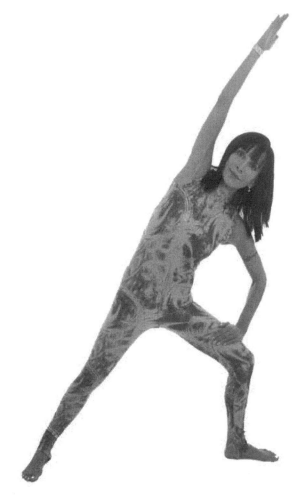

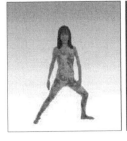 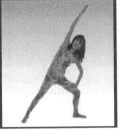 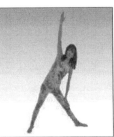 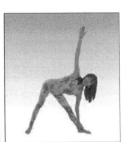

- Keeping your body still, simply bring your left arm straight up to the ceiling, the palm of your hand facing the front. Breathe in, and as you breathe out reach a little higher – as though you were trying to touch the ceiling with your fingertips. You should be aware of the extra stretch in the muscles surrounding your left shoulder – a great workout for these particular muscles, helping to keep your shoulders in correct alignment, and preventing rounding of the shoulders. Now slowly straighten your right leg.

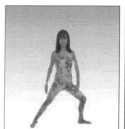
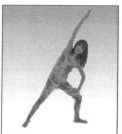
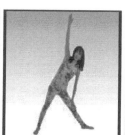
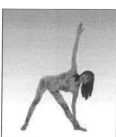

- Slowly and carefully, slide your right hand down towards your ankle. If you can't go that far down just go as far as you can comfortably manage. Take hold of your ankle – or shin if you can't reach your ankle – to support your bodyweight and take the strain off your spine.

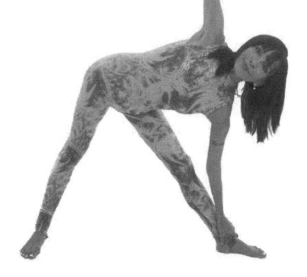

- You are now in the full *Triangle Pose*. Hold for at least 5 deep breaths.

Note: While holding *Triangle Pose*, continually press your tailbone out behind you, to keep your spine straight and long. Keep your left shoulder drawn back and your right shoulder forward, to ensure that your chest remains open and facing the front. Do not allow your chest to turn down to the floor.

Always support Triangle Pose by holding onto your supporting leg – to protect your lumbar spine muscles.

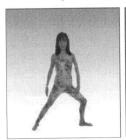 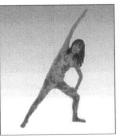 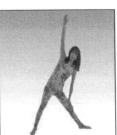 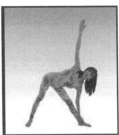

Reverse Triangle Pose

Reverse Triangle is performed from ***Triangle Pose:***

- Allow your right knee to bend again, and lower the right side of your body down to your thigh. You should now be close enough to the floor to enable you to place your right hand on the floor in front of your right instep. Make sure you keep your body facing forward at this stage. Hold for one deep breath.

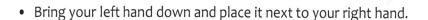

- Bring your left hand down and place it next to your right hand.

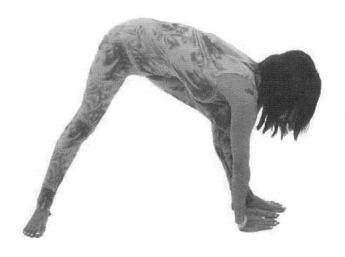

- Without allowing your left foot to swivel (it should stay exactly as it is), raise your right arm up towards the ceiling, turning your torso to face the other way.

- Focus on your shoulders – draw your right shoulder back and your left shoulder forward, to ensure as much turn in the torso as possible. Hold this pose for five breaths.

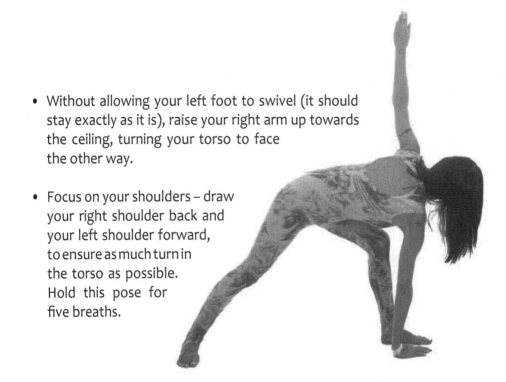

- Bring your right hand back down to the floor and turn your body to face the floor completely, and let your left heel lift. You should now have a hand either side of your right foot.

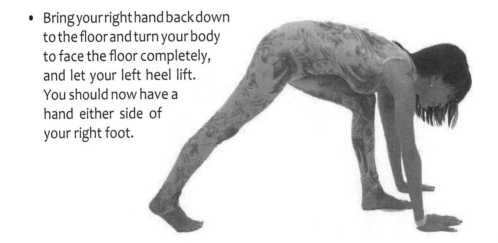

- Slide your left hand a little wider to the left, and take a big step forwards with your left foot, bringing both feet into line. Keeping your knees slightly bent, slowly uncurl, vertebra by vertebra, to standing position.

- Repeat *Triangle* and *Reverse Triangle* from the start, for the left side of your body.

Note: By not allowing your left foot to swivel as you go into Reverse Triangle, you turn your body from the hip instead, and this can ease stiffness and increase mobility in the hip joint.

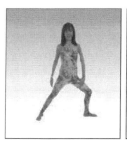 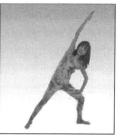 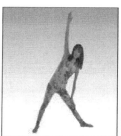 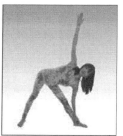

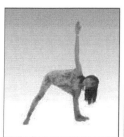 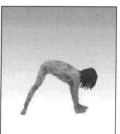 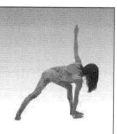 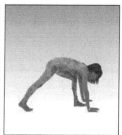

Warrior 1

*A fabulous energising pose with some strong proven clinical benefits: **Warrior 1** will boost the blood flow to and from the lower leg, significantly decreasing the risk of Deep Vein Thrombosis (DVT). **Warrior 1** can also help prevent varicose veins, by strengthening the valves of the leg veins. It is also a great strengthening and toning pose, especially for the thighs and hips.*

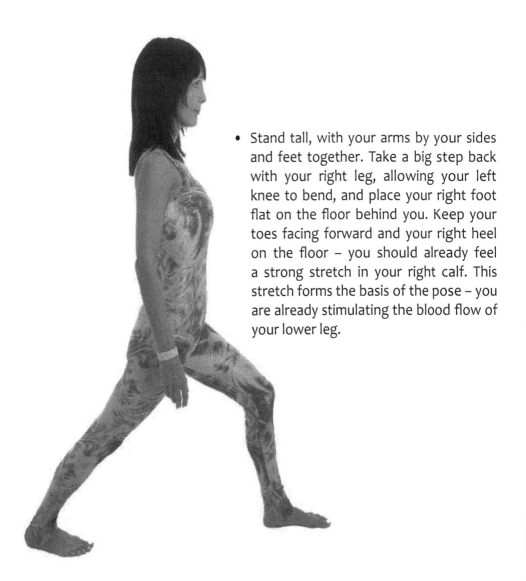

- Stand tall, with your arms by your sides and feet together. Take a big step back with your right leg, allowing your left knee to bend, and place your right foot flat on the floor behind you. Keep your toes facing forward and your right heel on the floor – you should already feel a strong stretch in your right calf. This stretch forms the basis of the pose – you are already stimulating the blood flow of your lower leg.

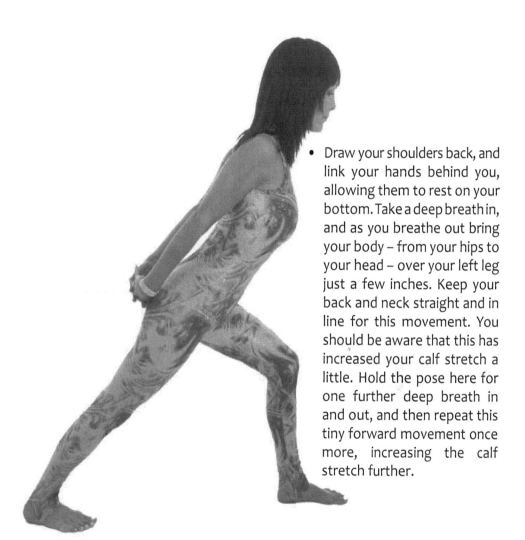

- Draw your shoulders back, and link your hands behind you, allowing them to rest on your bottom. Take a deep breath in, and as you breathe out bring your body – from your hips to your head – over your left leg just a few inches. Keep your back and neck straight and in line for this movement. You should be aware that this has increased your calf stretch a little. Hold the pose here for one further deep breath in and out, and then repeat this tiny forward movement once more, increasing the calf stretch further.

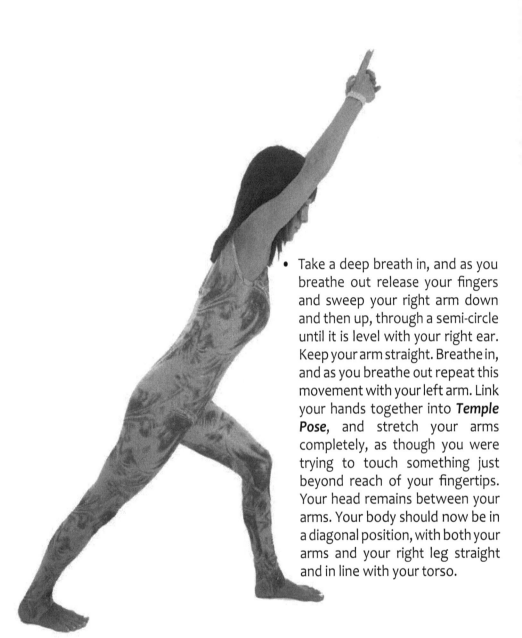

- Take a deep breath in, and as you breathe out release your fingers and sweep your right arm down and then up, through a semi-circle until it is level with your right ear. Keep your arm straight. Breathe in, and as you breathe out repeat this movement with your left arm. Link your hands together into **Temple Pose**, and stretch your arms completely, as though you were trying to touch something just beyond reach of your fingertips. Your head remains between your arms. Your body should now be in a diagonal position, with both your arms and your right leg straight and in line with your torso.

- Hold the pose for 3 deep breaths, and then start to bend your left knee and, slowly, bring your arms and body forwards and down, until you can place your hands on the floor underneath your shoulders. Try to keep your arms and back straight, and stretch as you come down – this movement should come from the hips.

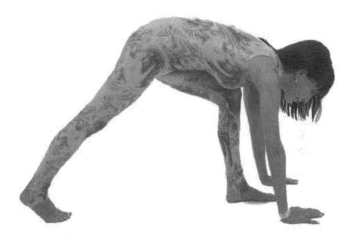

- Now, lift your right heel and slide or step back with your right foot as far as possible, allowing your left knee to bend more to accommodate this movement. You should now feel a strong stretch in the pelvic/groin area and running down the front of your right thigh. Hold this stretch for 3 deep breaths, your bodyweight supported by your arms.

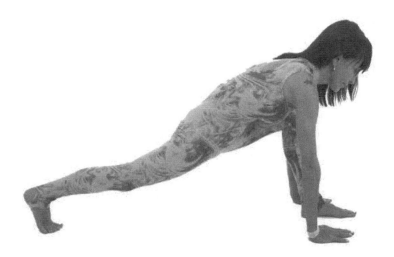

- Very gently place your right knee down onto the floor – make sure it is well cushioned with your yoga mat or folded towel. You are now in a "lunge" position, with your right leg stretched out behind you, and your bodyweight on your left leg and both arms.

From here, making sure you keep your bodyweight on your left leg (i.e. don't push back onto your right knee), lift your chest off your left thigh and bring your body into an upright position. Maintain your lunge position, trying to keep your right thigh drawn down towards the floor. Bring your hands into **Prayer Pose**.

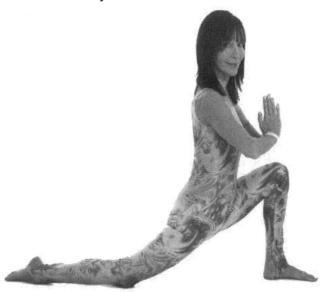

- Hold for a minimum of 3 deep breaths – during which time you will be aware of the very strong stretch this pose produces in the pelvic area and extended thigh.

- You have now completed **Warrior 1** pose.

- To come out of the pose, return your hands to the floor, tuck the toes of your right foot, lift your knee and step forwards, bringing both feet together. Keeping your knees slightly bent, uncurl slowly to standing.

- **Now repeat *Warrior 1* from the start, stepping back with your left leg.**

Note: This is a particularly strong stretch for the calves, thighs and pelvic area and, with regular practice, will increase your flexibility considerably.

Warrior 2

*Warrior 2 is a progression from **Warrior 1**, and is a fantastic strengthening and toning workout for the thighs. It brings a lot of power into the legs, so a great pose for runners and sports people in particular. Be warned – this is a tough pose to perform, and should be attempted only once you are comfortable with **Warrior 1**.*

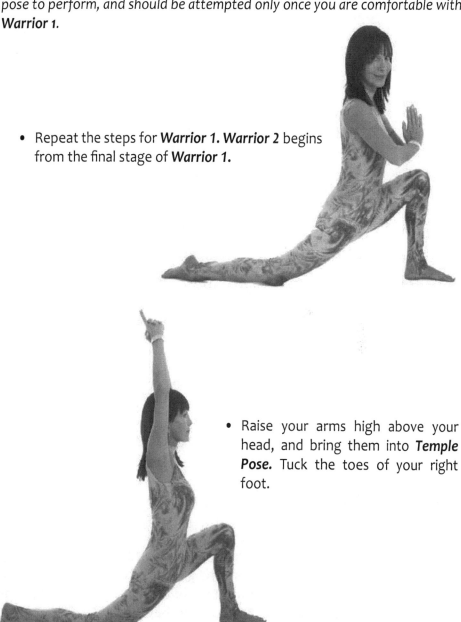

- Repeat the steps for **Warrior 1. Warrior 2** begins from the final stage of **Warrior 1.**

- Raise your arms high above your head, and bring them into **Temple Pose.** Tuck the toes of your right foot.

- Now, without changing the position of your left leg – it remains just as it is – simply straighten out your right leg. This will lift your right knee off the floor, and bring you into *Warrior 2.*

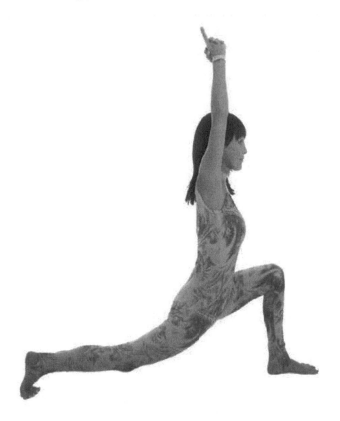

- Hold your completed pose for a minimum of 3 deep breaths, and then slowly stretch forward and down with your arms and your body, returning your hands to the floor underneath your shoulders. To finish, step your right foot forwards, bringing your feet together, and uncurl slowly to standing.

- **Repeat with your left leg.**

Note: **Your aim is to straighten your back leg without changing the position of your front leg - don't "push" yourself up with your front leg. Your body should remain at the same height throughout this movement. Keep your body upright, with your shoulders back and head up. The closer your back thigh is to the floor, the better.**

Proud Warrior

*A beautiful energising and strengthening pose. Thousands of years ago, **Proud Warrior** was used to "impress and intimidate our enemies" ..... Now, we use it to strengthen our shoulders and thighs, and to bring a sense of calm and tranquillity to the mind.*

- Stand with your legs wide apart – at least one metre - with your toes turned forward. Take a deep breath in, and as you breathe out lift your arms straight out to each side until they are level with your shoulders, with your palms facing the floor. Imagine someone pulling each of your hands, so you feel the stretch in your arms and shoulders.

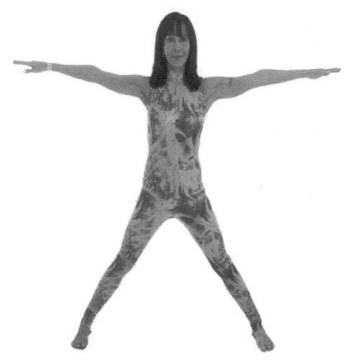

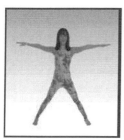 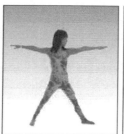 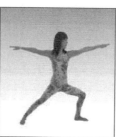 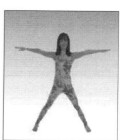

- Now, turn the toes of your right foot out to the side (90 degrees) – try to keep your right hip facing the front. With your next breath out, turn your head sideways to the right, aiming to position your chin directly over your right shoulder. Take care not to tip your head backwards.

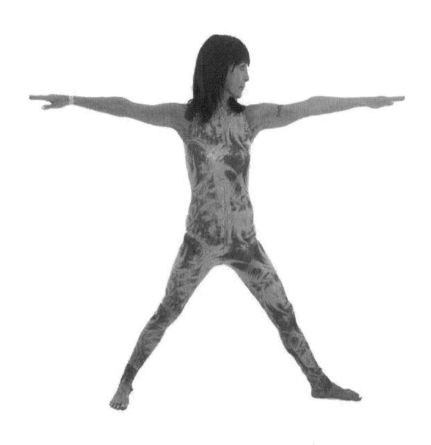

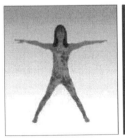 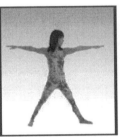 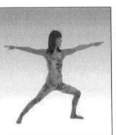 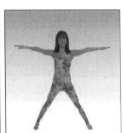

- Finally, breathe in and as you breathe out bend your right knee and bring your bottom down towards the floor, coming into a deep lunge position. You are now in **Proud Warrior.** Hold the pose for 5 deep breaths.

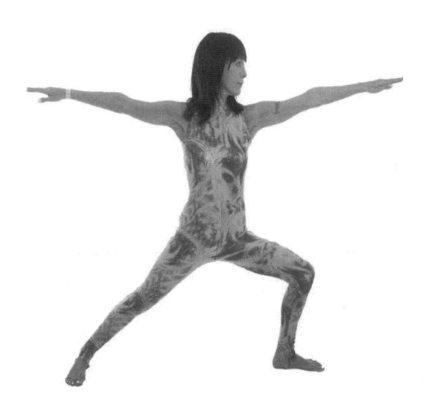

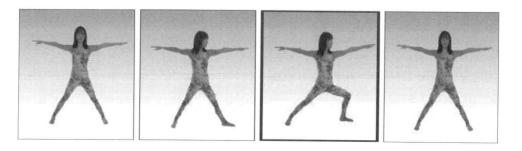

- Then, keeping your arms outstretched, slowly straighten your right leg, and return your head and your right foot to face the front.

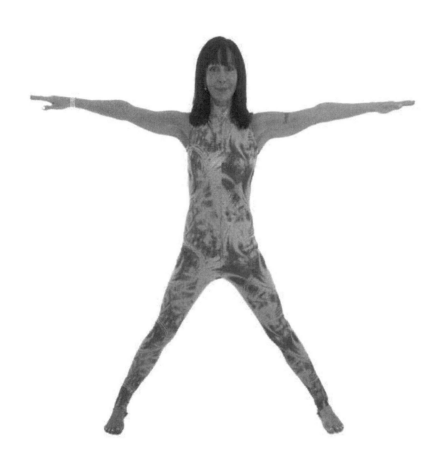

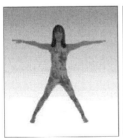
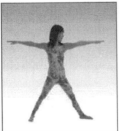
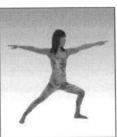
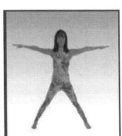

- Without relaxing your arms, turn the toes of your left foot out to the side, and repeat the above points but this time turning your head to the left and lunging with your left leg. Again, hold the pose for 5 deep breaths.

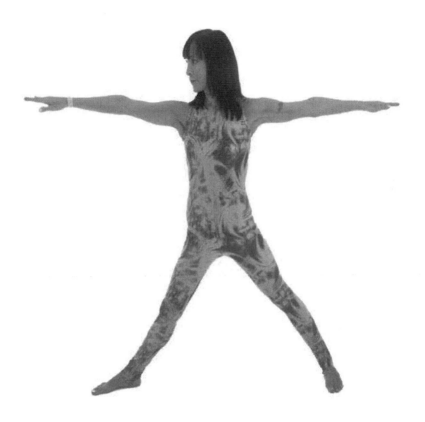

Note: Keep your shoulders relaxed, and your tailbone tucked under throughout the pose. Try to maintain the deep lunge position – it's easy to start straightening up without realising.

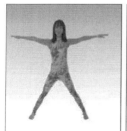 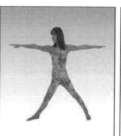 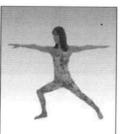 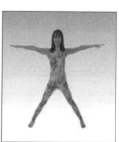

Assisted Side-Angle Pose

Assisted Side-Angle Pose is a close relative of both Triangle and Proud Warrior. It is a gentle and effective energising pose, and is considered to be a particularly good work-out for the heart – which is a muscle, after all. It will also strengthen the shoulders and hips.

- Repeat the first stage of **Proud Warrior.**

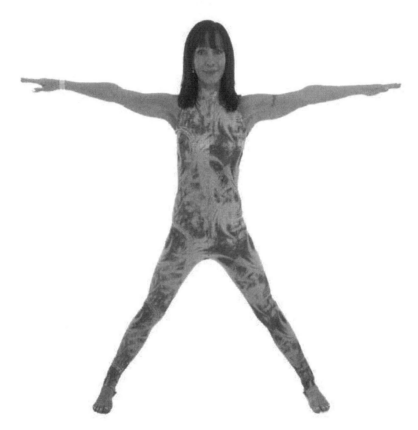

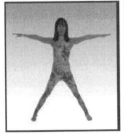 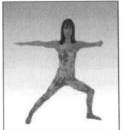 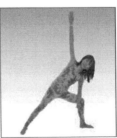 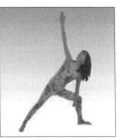

- Turn the toes of your right foot out to the side, clench your right fist, and bend your arm in at a 90 degree angle, with your forearm in a horizontal position. Now bend your right knee, dropping into a lunge position.

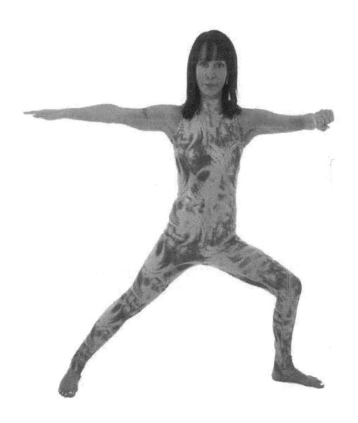

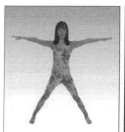 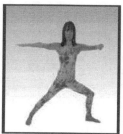 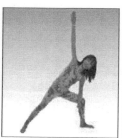 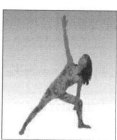

- Take a deep breath in and as you breathe out lean over from the waist, until you can rest your right forearm on your right thigh. Your left arm continues straight up until your fingertips face the ceiling, with your palm facing forwards. Take 3 deep breaths.

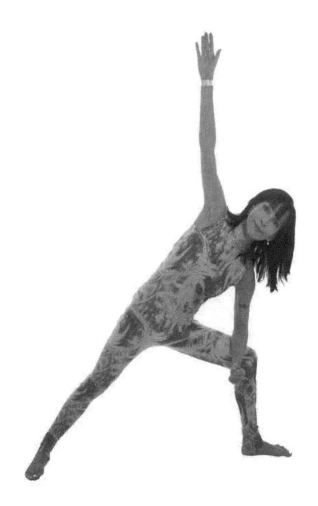

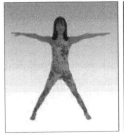 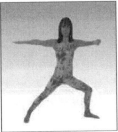 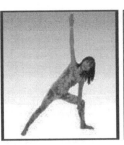 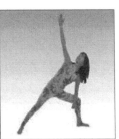

- Turn your head sideways to look up at the ceiling, and take two further breaths in and out.

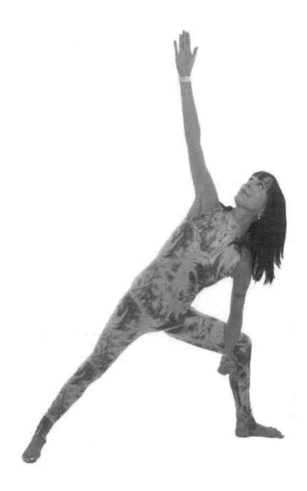

- Return your head to a forward position. Take another 3 deep breaths.

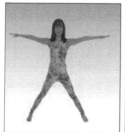 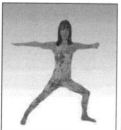 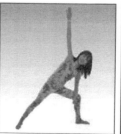 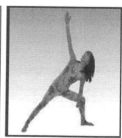

- You have now completed *Assisted Side-Angle Pose*. Slowly return your body to its upright position, with both arms outstretched to the sides. Straighten your right leg and turn your toes forward.

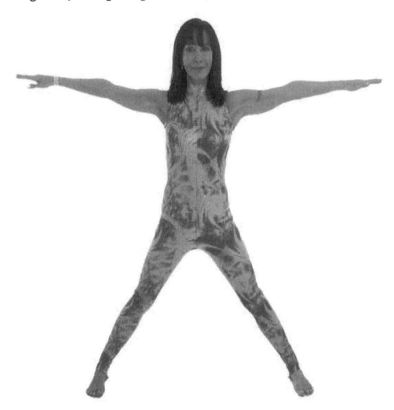

- Still with your arms outstretched, turn the toes of your left foot to the side and repeat the pose with your left knee bent and right arm raised.

Note: If the neck turns in this pose feel uncomfortable, simply leave them out and keep your face to the front throughout the pose.

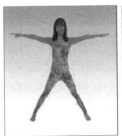 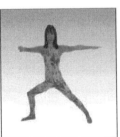 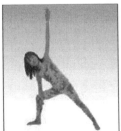 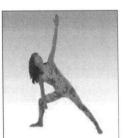

Modified Half-Candle Pose

Poor circulation is a common complaint, but it can be improved. Inactivity is the main culprit, so it is vital that you keep as active and mobile as possible. Prolonged periods of sitting slows the circulation down – this means cold hands and feet, puffy swollen ankles, and it can also affect your mental attitude, making you feel sluggish and apathetic. Inactivity can also increase the possibility of blood clots in the lower legs, leading to deep vein thrombosis.

Modified Half-Candle pose *helps to maintain healthy circulation to the legs. It stimulates lymphatic drainage, helping to remove excess fluid (oedema) from the ankles. It also helps prevent varicose veins, as it exercises the valves in the main leg veins, stimulating and strengthening the blood flow to the legs.*

- Lie on your back, with your knees bent, feet flat on the floor and your arms resting down by your sides.

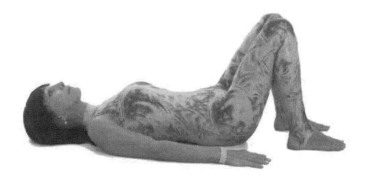

- Raise your right leg up towards the ceiling, keeping it as straight and as high as possible. Point your toes, feeling a stretch along the front of your foot.

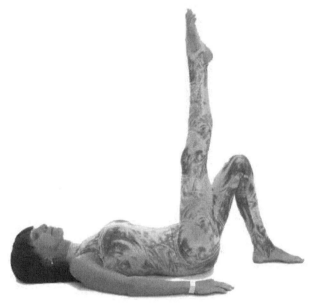

- Now flex your foot by drawing your toes down towards you and pressing your heel upwards (you should feel the stretch in your calf muscle when you do this).

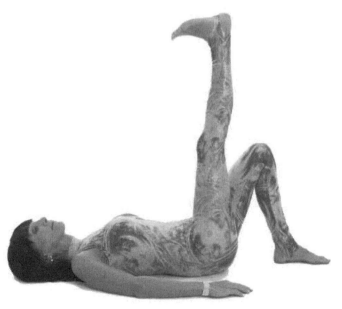

- Repeat this "point-flex" movement with your foot, keeping your leg as still as possible, until you have done ten of each. This movement is done quite quickly.

- Now, start to rotate your ankle, "drawing" a big circle with your toes, keeping the rest of your leg as still as possible. Do this slowly, stretching your foot all the way around your circle. Draw 4 circles in one direction, and then 4 circles the other way. Repeat this, so that you have drawn sixteen circles in total.

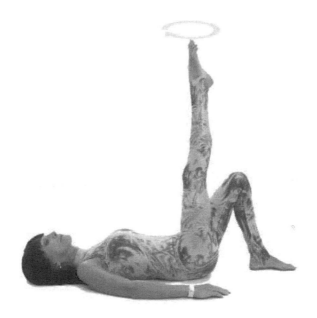

- Finally, repeat the "point-flex" movement once more, again doing ten of each. After this, bend your knee and take your foot back down to the floor.

- To complete the pose, raise your left leg to the ceiling, and repeat.

Note: Holding your leg up in the air is tiring and you will feel your lower leg aching a little. This is normal. Persevere though, as it makes the circulation work so much harder, and ensures that the valves in the leg veins are getting a good workout. Try not to let your leg "drift" down towards the floor during the pose.

Bridge Pose

*I try to include **Bridge** in every yoga class I teach, because of its amazing benefits – both physically and medically.*

*Physically, **Bridge** strengthens the muscles of the abdomen, lower back, bottom and thighs, and also ensures that the spine is able to flex and bend the way it was designed to.*

The medical benefits include:

1. *The easing of digestive problems – from relatively minor complaints such as indigestion, heartburn and acid reflux, to the more serious complaints like colitis and IBS (Irritable Bowel Syndrome)*
2. *It can reduce menstrual and pre-menstrual symptoms, especially cramps and associated back-ache.*
3. *It can also reduce menopausal and peri-menopausal symptoms, such as temperature fluctuations.*
4. *The pose stimulates the thyroid gland, which is located at the base of your throat, and helps to control your metabolism. So, if you think your metabolism is a little sluggish, this pose could be invaluable.*
5. *Finally, **Bridge** is a "mood elevator" pose – it works on the nervous system and has been shown to lift the spirits and ease depression by stimulating the production of Serotonin – known as your body's own "natural anti-depressant".*

- **Bridge Pose** is performed lying on your back, with your arms down by your sides, palms facing down. Your knees should be bent, feet flat on the floor. Feet and knees should be the same width as your hips.

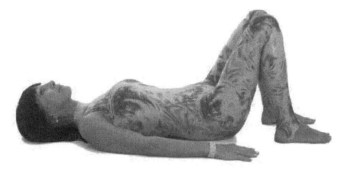

- Slowly, start to lift your bottom off the floor, raising your back, with your hips aimed up towards the ceiling. Walk your feet in a few steps towards your bottom and continue to raise your back, **lifting to your highest comfortable point**. Your arms remain relaxed and resting on the floor at your sides. Alternatively, you can link your fingers together and, keeping your arms straight, rest them on the floor directly underneath your back. **Do not try to wedge your hands into the small of your back – this is commonly seen, but it is not necessary, and you run the risk of damaging your wrists.**

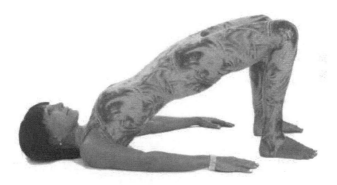

- When you have reached your comfortable height, hold your body still and focus on your breathing. Breathe in slowly, letting your abdomen rise and completely fill with air. Then, as you slowly breathe out, use your abdominal muscles to flatten the area down. Continue this slow breathing pattern, allowing the abdomen to rise and fall, for at least two minutes. You can hold the pose for up to 4 minutes if you feel comfortable!

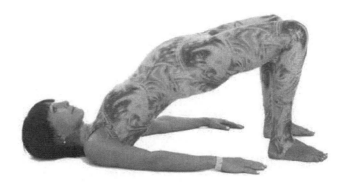

- When you are ready to come out of **Bridge Pose**, bring your arms back out to your sides on the floor if you have your hands linked underneath your back. Very slowly, return your body to the floor, letting your upper back meet the floor first and coming down through your spine, vertebra by vertebra, until your bottom finally touches down. Take your time with your descent – imagine you are working in slow motion, keep your back rounded, and bring each vertebra, one at a time, down to the floor.

- To finish, pull your knees into your chest and hug them tightly, using both arms. This protects the spine by stretching it in the opposite way to **Bridge Pose** – known as a "counter-stretch" - and is a very important part of the pose. Hold this stretch for at least thirty seconds.

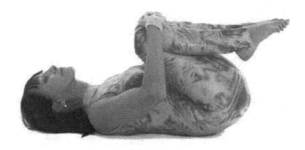

Note: Try to keep your Bridge at its original height throughout the pose – it is very easy to start drifting down to the floor without realising!

Windbreaker Pose

This is another great pose with medical benefits – and as the name might suggest, the benefits focus on the digestive system!

*Physically, **Windbreaker Pose** will stretch the muscles of the legs, loosen stiff hips and strengthen the abdominal, upper back, shoulder and neck muscles.*

*Medically, this pose can help to ease many common digestive problems – from relatively minor disorders such as indigestion, trapped wind and constipation, to more serious disorders like IBS (Irritable Bowel Syndrome) and Colitis, as **Windbreaker Pose** can help to relax the muscles that tend to spasm, causing pain and discomfort. Importantly, it can help to control and lessen stress, which is a recognised antagonist of disorders like these.*

***Windbreaker Pose** stimulates digestive transit, and it is therefore an important pose for eaters of red meat, which is known to slow the digestive process down and can 'clog up' the system.*

*In **Windbreaker Pose**, the digestive tract is divided in half length-wise, and you work on one half at a time. By working one side of the digestive tract while simultaneously allowing the other side to relax and lengthen, a "vacuum effect" is created by the deep yogic breathing. This stimulates the digestive process and gently "pushes" through the system anything that might be stuck or a little "sluggish" - be it trapped air, or digested food waste – and helps it on its way! Think of the way a sink plunger unblocks a sink by creating a vacuum - not a very pleasant analogy, but it does illustrate the point!*

- Lie on your back, with your arms down by your sides, legs stretched out and take a moment to relax your body, and slow down your breathing. Bend your right knee and draw it towards you. Clasp your hands around your knee, and "hug" it in as close to your chest as possible. Your left leg remains relaxed and on the floor.

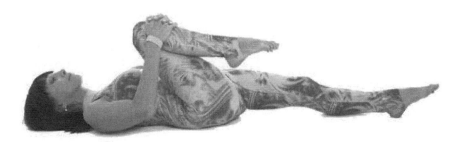

- Take a deep, slow breath in, and as you breathe out lift your head, shoulders and upper body off the floor, aiming to bring your chest and thigh as close together as possible.

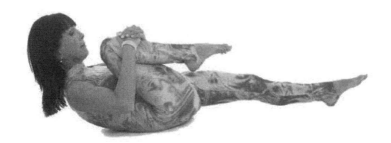

- Hold the pose for a minimum of 5 deep breaths, concentrating on breathing slowly and fully, inflating your lungs as fully as possible. Each time you breathe in, try to expand your rib cage, and press your abdomen to your thigh. Each time you breathe out flatten your abdomen, drawing your navel down towards your spine.

- On completion of your 5 deep breaths, breathe out as you gently lower your body back down to the floor. Release your leg and return it to the floor.

- Relax for 30 seconds, roll your head from side to side to release any tension and then repeat the pose with your left leg.

Note: You will find it difficult to breathe in deeply, as you have constricted one side of your body with your leg, making it harder for your lung on that side to inflate. Don't worry; this is normal, and an integral part of the pose.

If you start to feel strain and discomfort in your neck and shoulders, gently allow your head to rest back onto the floor. As long as you continue to hug your knee as close to your body as possible, and maintain the breathing instructions, you will still be working towards the digestive benefits of this pose.

SECTION 2

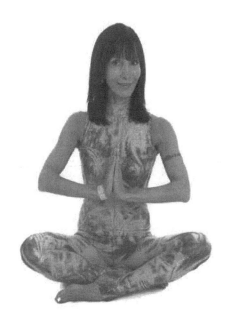

BALANCE POSES

BALANCE POSES

Yoga exercises unite mind and body, and balance plays an important part in this. Whenever we use our balance, we are improving our powers of concentration and our ability to focus.

There is also some evidence to show that using our balance on a regular basis can help us to retain our short term memory – which generally tends to fail us as we grow older.

Improving our balance will also make us steadier on our feet, and less prone to trips and falls.

The poses in this section will test and exercise your balance.

Heel to Toe Pose

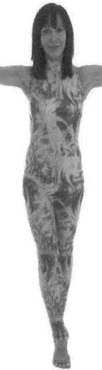

- Stand tall and place one foot directly in front of the other – your heels touching the toes behind, and both feet facing forwards. Take your arms straight out to your sides until they are at shoulder level, bringing you into a "T" shape – keep your arms straight, with your palms facing the floor. Make sure you are totally upright and not leaning forwards or backwards, and that your tailbone remains tucked under – it's very easy to stick your bottom out in this pose, so keep a check on this!

- When you have checked your posture is correct, all that remains to bring you into this pose is to close your eyes! By closing your eyes you are taking away a vital component of balance – your vision. You are stopping the signal from your eyes to your brain to keep you upright, and by doing this, you make your brain work a lot harder to compensate! Try to hold the pose for 3-5 deep breaths. If you feel wobbly, open your eyes for a few seconds to steady yourself and then continue.

- Repeat with your other foot in front.

Crane Pose

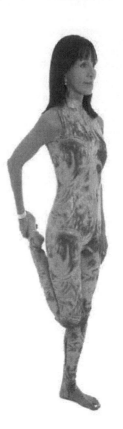

- Stand tall, with your feet together and your arms down by your side. Bend your right knee, lifting your foot up behind you, and take hold of your ankle (or the front of your foot) with your right hand. Gently pull back with your knee, bringing your thighs parallel and tuck your tailbone under so that you are not overly arching your back.

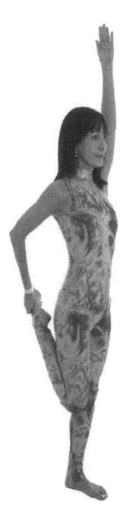

- Give yourself a few seconds to get your balance, and then raise your left arm directly up towards the ceiling, so that your arm is level with your ear. Keep your arm straight and high, look straight ahead, and hold the pose for 3-5 deep breaths.

- Repeat with your left leg.

Archer Pose

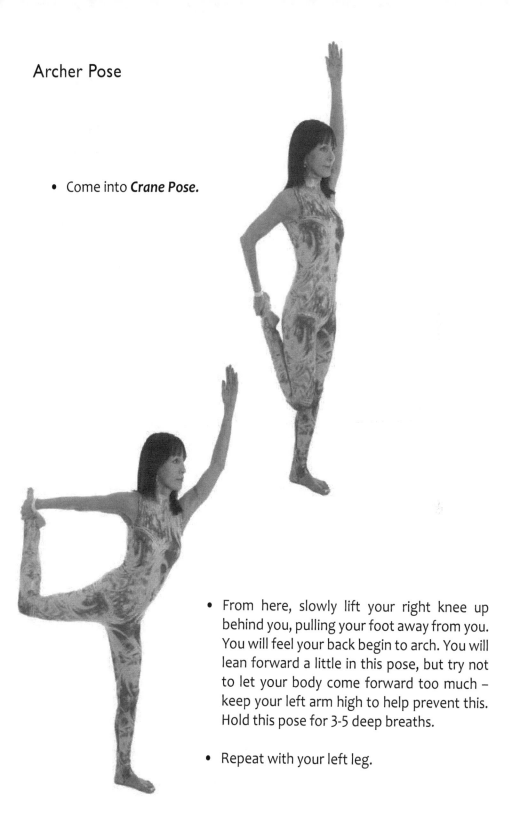

- Come into **Crane Pose.**

- From here, slowly lift your right knee up behind you, pulling your foot away from you. You will feel your back begin to arch. You will lean forward a little in this pose, but try not to let your body come forward too much – keep your left arm high to help prevent this. Hold this pose for 3-5 deep breaths.

- Repeat with your left leg.

Dart Pose

- Stand tall, with your feet together and place your hands on your hips. Step your right foot back, coming onto the toes of your right foot.

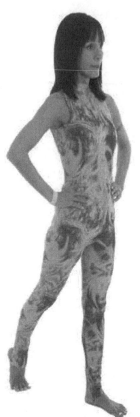

- Very slowly, lift your right foot off the floor and, keeping your leg straight, lift your leg up behind you while at the same time bringing your body down towards the floor. The aim of this pose is to keep a straight line running through the body, from the top of your head to the toes of your right foot. A slight bend on your supporting knee is recommended.

- Hold for 3-5 deep breaths.

- To work a little harder, you may now take your hands off your hips and extend your arms out in front of you, keeping them straight, either side of your head, and your hands in **Temple Pose**. This is an "optional extra", and should only be added when you can comfortably hold **Dart Pose** with your hands on your hips.

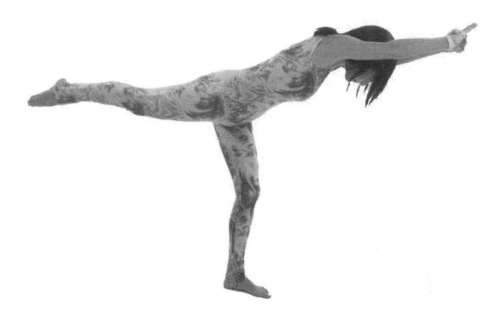

- Repeat with your left leg.

Note: The ultimate aim of *Dart Pose* is to bring yourself into a perfect horizontal line with your body and leg. However, this is not strictly necessary – as long as you maintain the straight line with your leg and body, you can lift your foot to whatever height you feel comfortable with – which may be just a few inches off the floor at first. If your foot is off the floor, you are using your balance!

Tree Pose

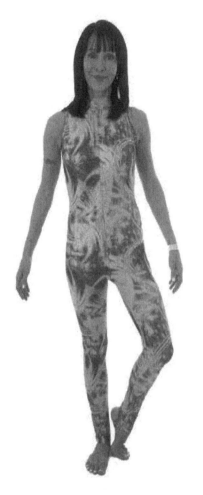

- Stand tall, with your feet together and your arms down by your side. Bend your right knee and turn your leg out to the side, without lifting your foot off the floor.

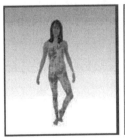 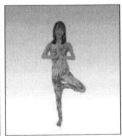 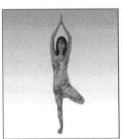 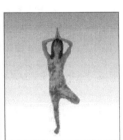

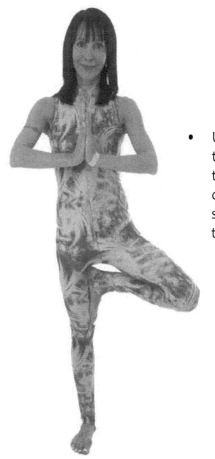

- Using your hand to help you if you wish, take the sole of your foot as high to the inside of your left thigh as you can comfortably manage. Give yourself a few seconds to get your balance here, and then place your hands in **Prayer Pose**.

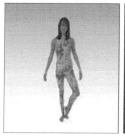 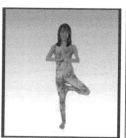 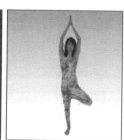 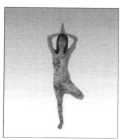

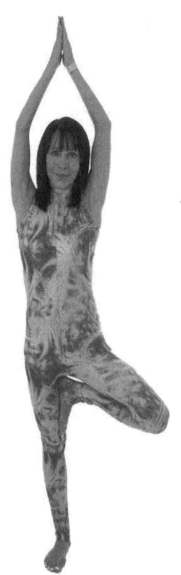

- When you are ready, take a deep slow breath in while you raise your arms high above your head – keeping your hands in **Prayer Pose** (you may cross your thumbs over each other to help keep your hands together).

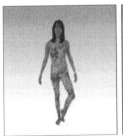 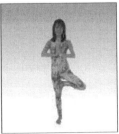 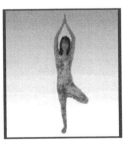 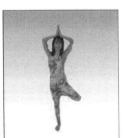

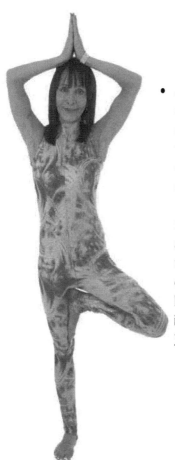

- As you breathe out, slowly bend your elbows out to each side and bring your hands – still in *Prayer Pose* - down until your wrists rest on the top of your head. Your elbows should remain drawn out to each side, with your fingertips still facing upward.

Stand still and upright, keeping your body tall, and focus on your breathing – allowing your ribcage to expand as you breathe in, and contracting your abdominal muscles as you breathe out. Make sure that you do not "sink" into your left hip. Hold this position for 3-5 deep breaths.

- To finish, as you breathe in raise your arms high, with your hands still in *Prayer Pose*, stretching to your fullest height, and as you breathe out release your hands and bring your arms down to your sides.

- Repeat with your left leg.

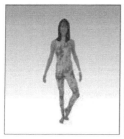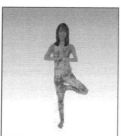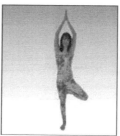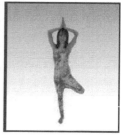

Eagle Pose

- Stand tall, with your feet a few inches apart, knees slightly bent and your arms by your sides. Bring your arms straight out in front of you to shoulder level, with your palms facing inwards. Now bend your elbows, bringing your fingertips up to face the ceiling, and bring your arms together. Your arms should now be at a 90 degree angle at the elbow.

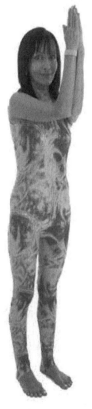

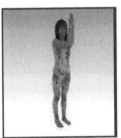 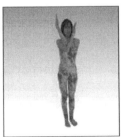 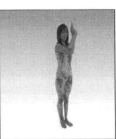 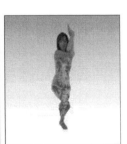

- Lift your right elbow and cross it over the left, and then "wind" your forearms around each other, and try to bring your hands into **Prayer Pose**. Don't worry if you cannot manage this - just go as far as you can.

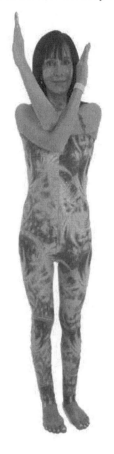

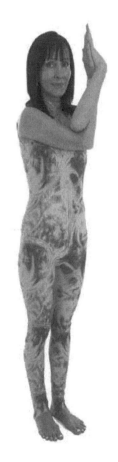

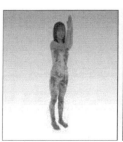 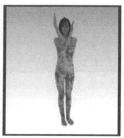 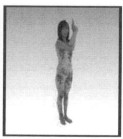 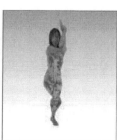

- Now, increase the bend on your knees, lift your right foot off the floor and cross your right thigh over your left. Try to "tuck" your toes behind your left calf. (Again, don't worry if you can't quite manage this – as long as you have one foot off the floor you are using your balance.)

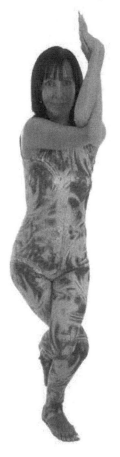

- Hold the pose for 3-5 breaths and then repeat with your left arm and leg crossed over.

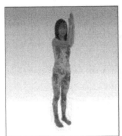 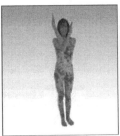 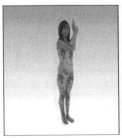 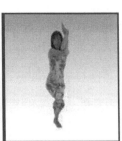

Standing Half Lotus Pose

- Stand tall, bend your right knee and turn your knee out.

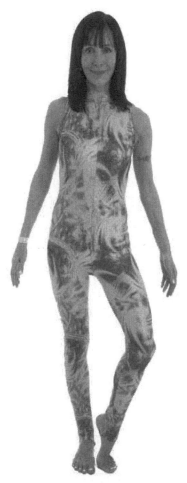

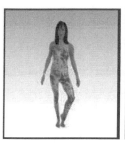 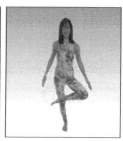 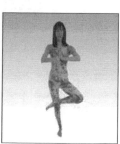 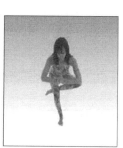

- Lift your right foot off the ground and cross your ankle over your left thigh just above the knee. Your right knee should be facing out to the right-hand side, and your left knee should now be slightly bent

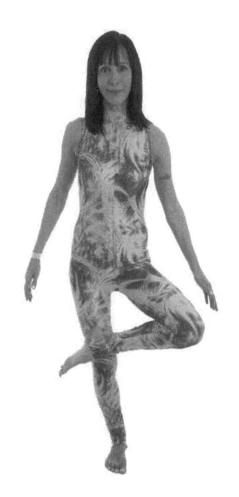

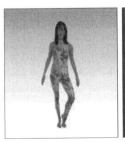 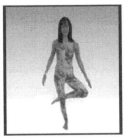 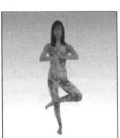 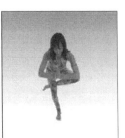

- Give yourself a few seconds to get your balance here, and then bring your hands into **Prayer Pose.**

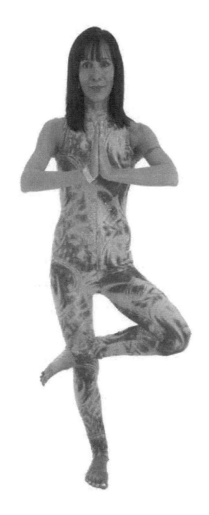

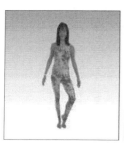 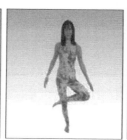 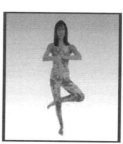 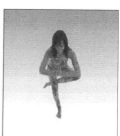

- Now increase the bend on your left knee, and start to bend forwards from the hips – pressing your tailbone out behind you, and keeping your shoulders back. Try to keep your back straight, and your neck in line with your spine.

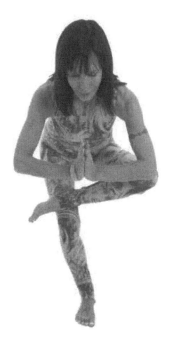

- Hold the pose for 3-5 breaths before slowly straightening up and releasing your leg.

- Repeat with your left leg crossed over your right.

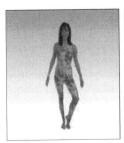 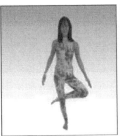 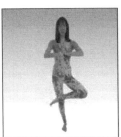 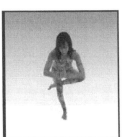

Kneeling Crescent Moon Pose

This balancing pose also uses the core stability muscles – so you may be aware of some involuntary muscle tremor from the core area of your body. Just focus on your breathing and it will slowly lessen.

- Come onto your hands and knees – your hands should be under your shoulders with your fingers facing forwards, and knees directly under your hips. Keep your neck in line with your spine – so you are looking down at the floor. Make sure that you do not tuck your toes.

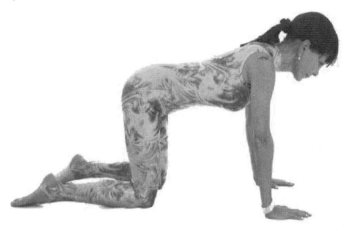

- Raise your right arm up until it is at ear level, the palm of your hand facing the floor. Keep your arm straight. Now extend your right leg out behind you, lifting it up until it is level with your body. Keep your leg straight, with your knee facing the floor.

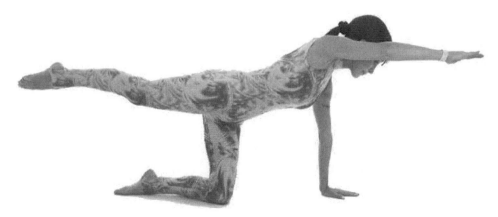

- When you feel ready, turn your body to your right-hand side, raising your arm as you do so, until your fingers are pointing to the ceiling. Your right leg will also turn, and remains in line with your body.

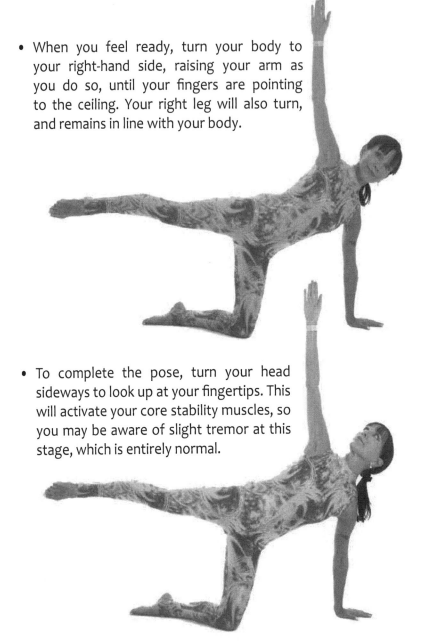

- To complete the pose, turn your head sideways to look up at your fingertips. This will activate your core stability muscles, so you may be aware of slight tremor at this stage, which is entirely normal.

- Hold this pose for approximately 3 breaths, and then repeat with your left arm and leg.

Note: While in this pose, do not tuck the toes of your supporting foot. While this may make the pose easier to hold, it stops the core stability muscles from working because you are stabilising yourself with your foot instead!

SECTION 3

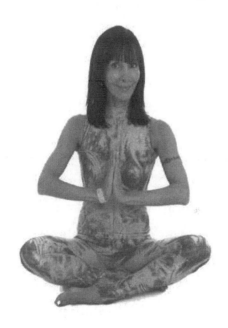

STRENGTHENING POSES

STRENGTHENING POSES

Strengthening poses require stamina and a strong will! The poses in this section will work your muscles hard without adding bulk – instead, as your muscles grow stronger, they will become longer and leaner. Your body will become more powerful, with firmer, more defined musculature.

Core stability muscles are featured heavily in this section. These muscles are located in the abdomen, buttocks, inner thighs and lower back, and are often referred to as your "girdle of strength" or "powerhouse". This area is your body's fulcrum of control, and it is very important to keep these muscles strong. They play an essential role as the main support system for the abdominal and pelvic area, enabling you to stand and move in the correct way. Strong core stability muscles will help to keep the body evenly balanced and aligned on both sides, thereby reducing the likelihood of back, shoulder and hip problems.

Incline Plank Pose

A strong pose with many benefits, including:

- *The strengthening of the shoulder joints and the surrounding shoulder muscles*
- *The strengthening of the upper back muscles*
- *The strengthening and toning of the pectoral (chest wall) muscle*
- *The toning of the biceps and triceps (the muscles of the upper arms)*
- *The strengthening and toning of the abdominal and lower back muscles*

*In a nutshell, **Incline Plank** is a great pose to improve upper body strength and tone, with the added bonus of firming the abs!*

- Come onto your hands and knees. Ensure that your hands are directly underneath your shoulders with your fingers facing forward, and that your knees are together, and underneath your hips. Keep your neck long and in alignment with your spine. Your breathing throughout **Incline Plank** is long and slow, filling the lungs completely each time you breathe in, and emptying the lungs completely each time you breathe out. Tuck the toes of both feet under.

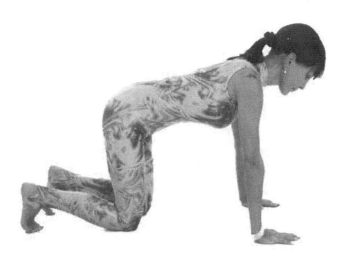

- Take a deep breath in and as you breathe out, slide your right foot away from you until your right leg is straight, toes remaining on the floor.

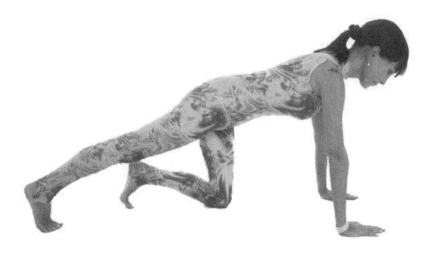

- With your next breath out, slide your left foot away until your feet are together behind you, and both legs are straight. You are now in *Incline Plank* pose – a straight line from head to toe.

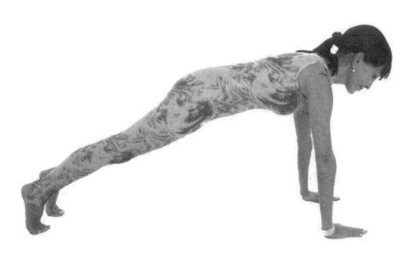

- Aim to hold the position for a slow count of ten. If this is too hard, aim initially for a count of five – you will soon be able to increase your holding time as you get stronger.

- When you are ready to come out of the pose, slowly bend your knees and replace them, **gently**, onto the floor. From here, come into **Child Pose** for up to one minute.

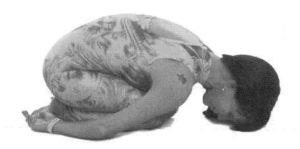

Note: In *Incline Plank* Pose your upper body and abdominal muscles work very hard indeed. Try to keep your breathing steady and slow, and resist the urge to hold your breath!

As you become stronger you can gradually increase the time you hold this pose – but bear in mind that technique is more important than timing, so work on achieving the perfect pose before trying to increase your timing. Remember, it is much better to perform a perfect Incline Plank for just ten seconds, than a less-than-perfect pose for twenty!

Side Incline Plank Pose

Side Incline Plank is a more advanced pose, and gives you a fantastic strengthening workout for your shoulders and upper arms. It also works the core stability muscles. **Side Incline Plank** should be seen as a progression from **Incline Plank,** and should not be done until **Incline Plank** can be performed with relative ease.

- **Side Incline Plank** is performed from **Incline Plank** position.

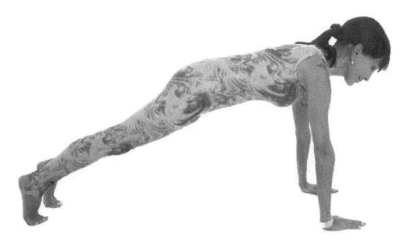

- From **Incline Plank,** lift your right foot and cross it over your left ankle – your toes should touch the floor on the other side.

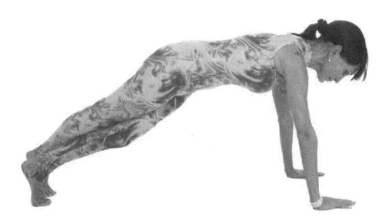

- Turn your body to the right, and lift your right arm straight up to the ceiling.

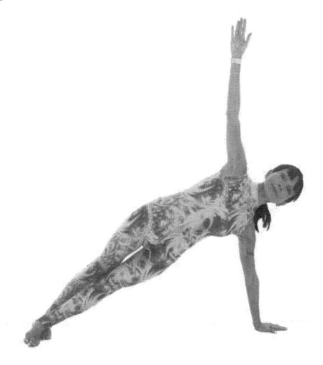

- To come out of the pose safely, bend your left knee and place it on the floor first, and then bring your right knee and right arm down so you are on all fours.

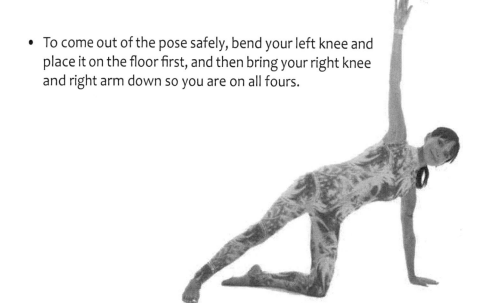

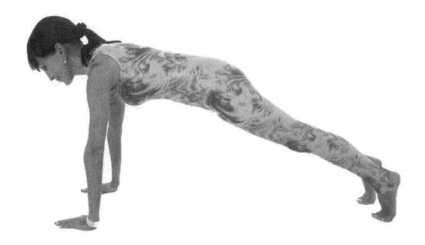

- Repeat to the other side.

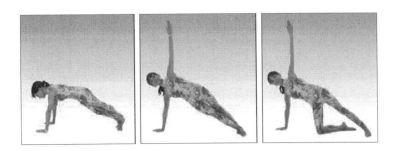

Note: When you can practice Side Incline Plank with relative ease and are ready to work a little harder, you may turn your head up to the ceiling during the final stage, to activate your core stability muscles.

A certain amount of pressure is placed on the wrists during the this pose, so it is recommended that you perform "Carpal Stretch" which can be found in the "Flexibility" section, directly after completing Side Incline Plank.

Scorpion Pose

Scorpion is a great strengthening pose for the upper body, giving you a very effective workout for your shoulders, upper arms and pectoral muscles.

- Come onto your hands and knees, placing your hands at shoulder height but wider than shoulder width, and your knees directly underneath your hips.

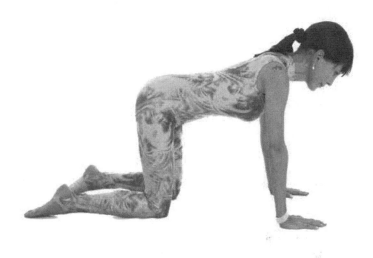

- Lift your right knee and extend your leg straight out behind you, raising it until it is level with your body.

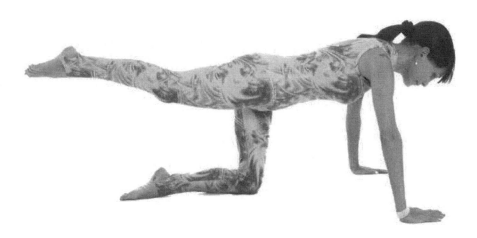

- Take more of your bodyweight onto your arms, by pushing forward slightly from your shoulders. Breathe in, and as you breathe out bend your elbows and lower your chest and your head down towards the floor – you are aiming to have your chest and your nose just an inch or so off the floor. Your elbows should be pointing to the ceiling. At the same time, raise your right leg up as high as you can, and to work even harder, push more of your bodyweight onto your arms until your elbows are directly over your wrists. Hold this position for 2 deep breaths.

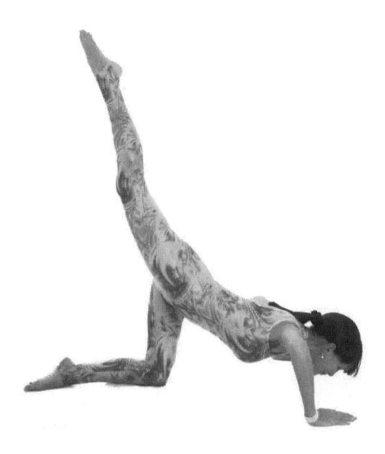

- Keeping your right thigh high and still, bend your right knee, and drop your heel down towards your bottom, with your foot flexed.

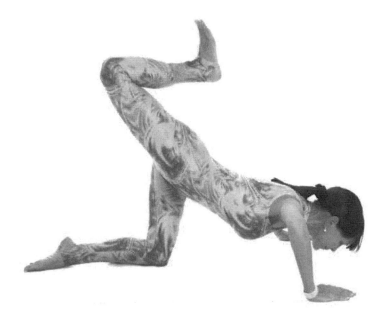

- You are now in the complete **Scorpion Pose**. Hold for a further 2 deep breaths, before slowly straightening your arms and returning your right knee to the floor.

- Repeat with your left leg.

Note: The more bodyweight on your arms, the harder you work and the better the results. However, this is a difficult pose to master, so increase the amount of bodyweight on your arms slowly, over a period of time.

"T"- Stand (Modified and Full)

T-Stand poses strengthen the shoulders and pectoral muscles, with the added bonus of a strong core stability workout. The modified version should be mastered before you attempt the full version.

Modified T- Stand:

- Come onto hands and knees, with your fingers facing forwards and your knees under your hips.

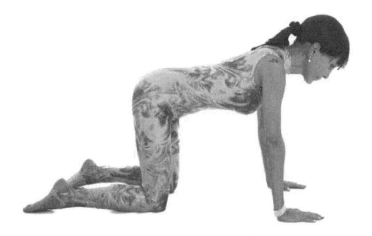

- Tuck under the toes of your right foot, and without lifting your foot off the floor slide it out behind you until your leg is straight.

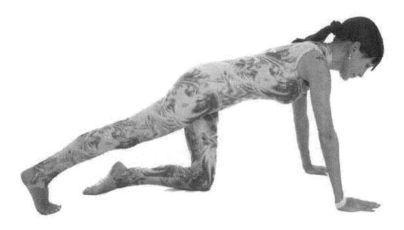

- Turn your body to the right, allowing your right foot to turn as well but keep the sole of your foot flat on the floor. Lift your right hand to the ceiling, and try to keep both arms in line (thus creating the "T" shape which gives this pose its name.)

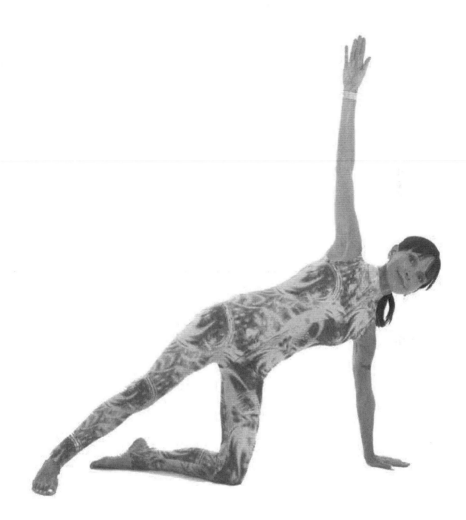

- To complete your **Modified T-Stand,** turn your head sideways to look straight up at the ceiling.

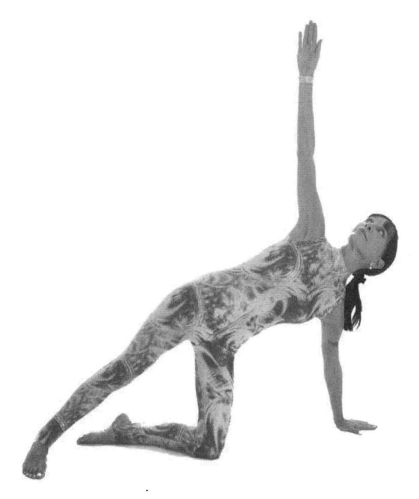

- Hold the pose for 3-5 deep breaths before gently returning to hands and knees.

- Repeat with your left arm and leg.

Note: Do not attempt the full T-Stand until you can do the modified version comfortably.

Full T- Stand:

- Repeat the steps for *Modified T-Stand.*

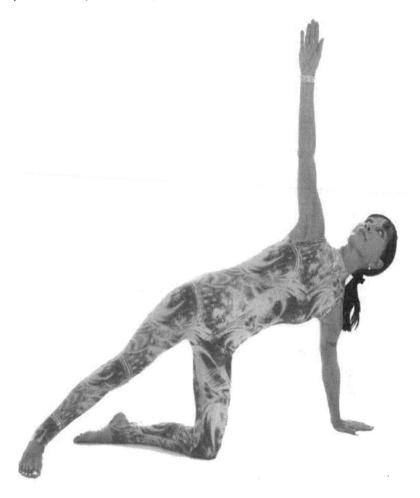

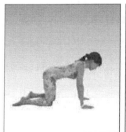 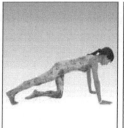 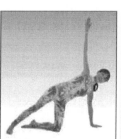 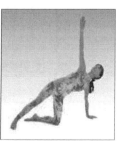

- From the final stage of **Modified T-Stand**, there is just one more movement to bring you into **Full T-Stand**: Lift your left knee off the floor, straighten your leg and hook your left foot behind your right ankle. At this stage, just your left hand and the sole of your right foot should be on the floor.

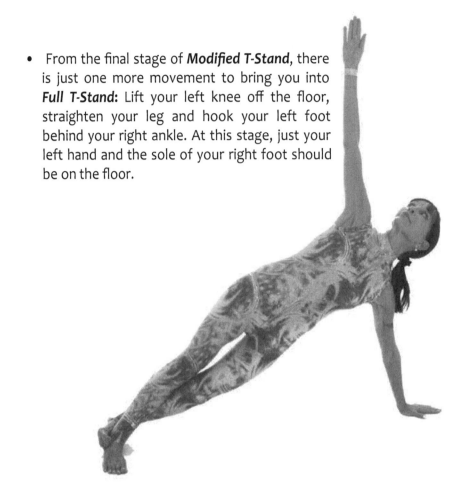

- Hold the pose for 3-5 deep breaths before gently returning to hands and knees.

- Repeat with your left arm and leg.

Note: The head turns in both Modified and Full T-Stand will cause your core stability muscles to work hard, and you will feel some tremor from the core area of your body as you try to keep your balance – particularly in the full pose. Be prepared!

As a certain amount of pressure is placed on the wrists during this pose, it is recommended that you perform "Carpal Stretch" which can be found in the "Flexibility" section, directly after completing Full T-Stand.

Moving Cobra Pose

Moving Cobra is a fabulous pose to strengthen the shoulders, upper arms and pectoral muscles. The pose is performed slowly, using discipline and control, and the strengthening benefits will be apparent almost from the start!

- From hands and knees, drop your bottom down to your heels, chest to thighs and forehead to floor. Your arms should be outstretched on the floor in front of you, with your hands slightly wider than shoulder-width.

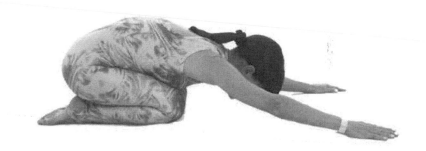

- Simultaneously, raise your head, and lift your bottom off your heels. Allow your elbows to bend now, and drop your chest right down towards the floor, aiming to come within an inch off the floor with your chest and face. At this stage, your bottom should be as high in the air as possible, and your elbows should be pointing to the ceiling. You should also be aware of a small arch in your lower back.

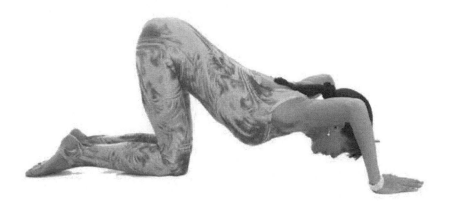

- As though in slow motion, start to move your body forward along the floor, travelling slowly and keeping as close to the floor as possible with your chest.

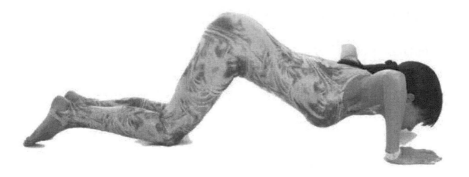

- Finally drop your hips as you come through your arms and into **Cobra Pose.** At this stage, your elbows should be slightly bent, shoulders dropped and relaxed, and your legs straight and together behind you.

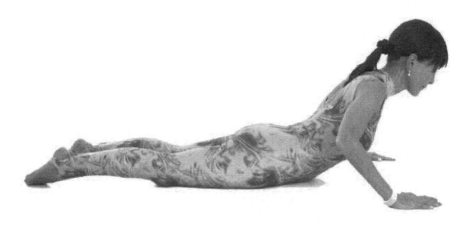

- Hold the pose for 3 deep breaths.

- Return to your starting position by using your arms to push back onto hands and knees, and dropping your bottom back down onto your heels. Your arms should once again be straight out in front of you.

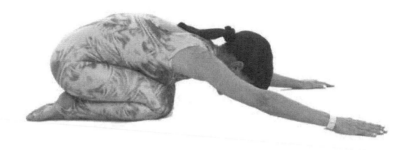

- Repeat *Moving Cobra* twice more.

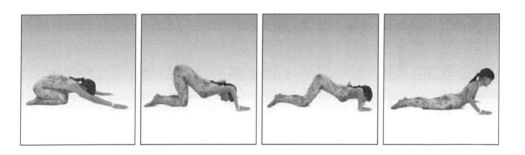

Note: Your hands should stay in exactly the same position throughout the pose. The slower you can perform Moving Cobra, the better!

"Z" Pose

A simple yet effective pose to strengthen and lengthen the thighs.

- Kneel on the floor and bring both arms straight out in front of you at shoulder level, palms facing the floor. Your feet should be flat behind you – don't tuck your toes under.

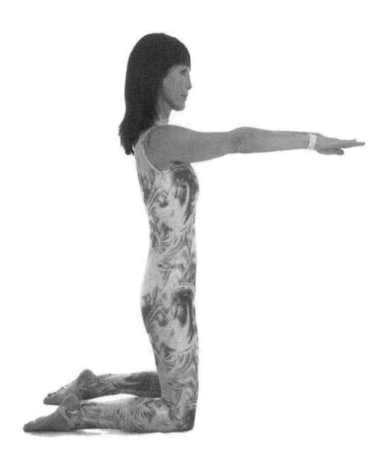

- Breathe in, and as you breathe out lean back in a straight line, going as far back as you can manage. You should feel a strong pull in your thighs.

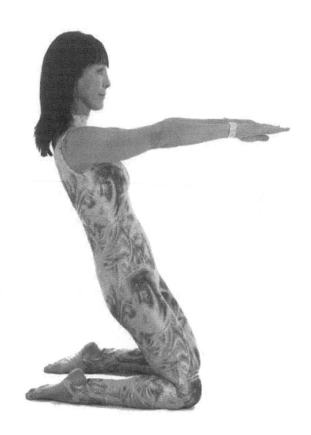

- Hold the pose for two breaths before returning to your starting position. Repeat the pose twice more.

Note: Your body should come into a "Z" position in this pose, so keep your arms straight and at shoulder length. Challenge yourself with this pose by trying to bring your body a little lower each time you repeat it.

Baby Crow Pose

Baby Crow is a fabulous workout for your feet – by using the stabilising muscles in your toes, you are strengthening both the toes and the arches of your feet. This is a particularly useful pose for people who run, walk or dance, and anyone who plays a lot of sports.

- From hands and knees, toes tucked under behind you, push yourself up onto your toes. With your fingertips on the floor to stabilise you, lift as high as you can onto your tip-toes, drawing your knees upwards, and at the same time bringing your body down slightly to meet your thighs.

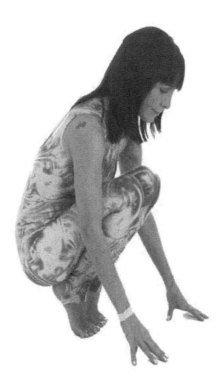

- Look at the floor in front of you, and give yourself a few seconds to become stable and balanced.

- When you are ready, lift your hands off the floor, turning your palms towards the ceiling and with your forearms parallel to the floor.

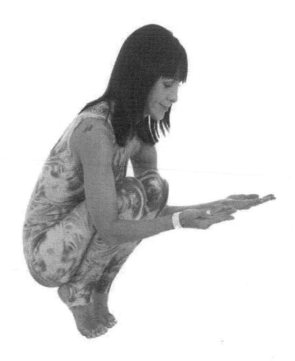

- Hold the pose for at least 6-8 breaths. You will feel a lot of "wobbling" and movement coming from your toes, and also from your ankles – the stabilising muscles in your toes and ankles are working overtime to keep you balanced, which in turn is strengthening the arches of your feet.

- When you are ready to come out of the pose, simply return your hands to the floor and uncurl slowly from there.

Note: During this pose, make sure your torso is leaning forward slightly, and not upright, to make the stabilising muscles work as hard as possible. This pose will also strengthen weak ankles.

Standalone Jack-knife Pose

This great pose concentrates on strengthening the core stability muscles and thighs. It is a difficult pose to master, but its strong benefits for the core stabilisers make it worth the effort! The main job of the core stability muscles is to support the core area of your body, taking away pressure on the spine and surrounding muscles caused by poor posture. This, in turn, will reduce your risk of developing a back problem.

- Sit on the floor on your mat, with your knees bent and your feet flat on the floor in front of you. Your feet and knees should be together, with your heels approximately 18 inches away from your bottom. At this point your back is likely to be slightly rounded. Hold underneath each knee with your hands, and straighten your back as much as you can, drawing your shoulders back and lengthening your neck.

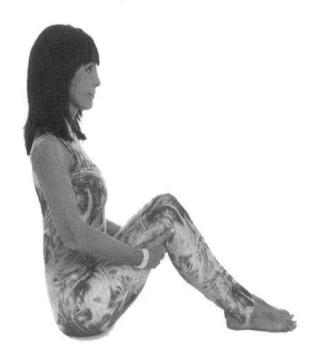

- Still holding under the knees, come onto your toes and "walk" your feet in a few inches closer. As you do this, you will start to lean back slightly – but make sure you keep your back straight. Now, when you feel ready, carefully lift your toes an inch off the floor, leaving you balancing on just your bottom.

- Allow yourself a few seconds to adjust to this stage, and then, very slowly, start to raise your feet up until your toes are level with your knees, calves parallel with the floor. As your feet slowly come up into this position, you will start to lean back a little more – which is fine – but make sure you are keeping your shoulders drawn back, to stop the spine from rounding.

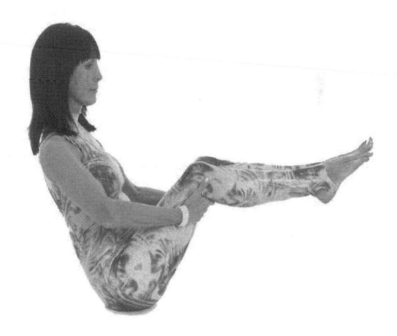

- At this point you may notice some involuntary shaking and tremor from your core – this is good news! Your core stability muscles are now working very hard. Keep your breathing slow and controlled, and try to hold the pose still for 3 deep breaths.

- Continue to hold under your knees, while you extend your legs – the ultimate aim of the pose is to come into a V shape, with your spine straight and your legs completely extended, but take your time to get to this level. Try a partial extension of your legs first, gradually working up to a complete extension in your own time. Release your legs, taking your arms straight out in front of you.

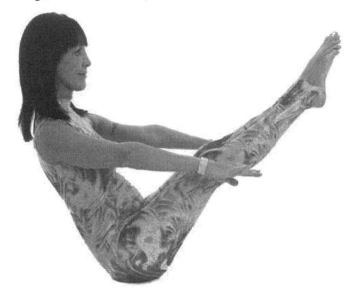

- You are now in *Standalone Jack-knife Pose*. Hold the pose for 5 deep breaths, concentrating on keeping your shoulders back and your spine straight.

- On completion of your breaths, take hold underneath your knees once more and slowly return your feet to the floor. Stretch your back by pushing your rib cage firmly to your thighs, with your shoulders back, to remove any tension from the spine.

Note: It is very important that you keep your back as straight as possible, with your shoulders drawn back, throughout this pose. It will be very tempting to let your back become rounded, so use your deep, yoga breathing to help you stay focussed!

Increase the length of time you hold the pose at your own pace. However, remember that technique is more important, so make sure that you perfect your pose before increasing your time. That means learning to hold the pose with a straight spine, shoulders back, a long neck, and with your legs completely extended.

Extended Bridge Pose

This pose is much harder than it looks! **Extended Bridge Pose** *is another wonderful workout for the core stability muscles. Remember, the stronger your core stability muscles, the less likely you are to have a problem with your back, hips or knees. Strong core stability muscles will also improve your posture and body alignment.*

- Lie on your back, with your arms down by your sides and your knees bent. Your feet and knees should be hip-width apart.

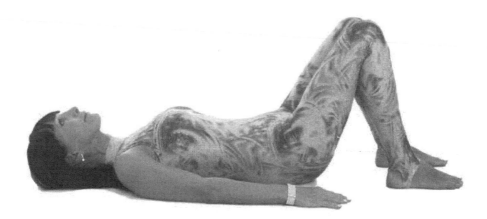

- Breathe in, and as you breathe out lift your bottom and your back off the floor until you are in a straight bridge position – that is, a straight line from your shoulders to your knees, with no arch in your spine.

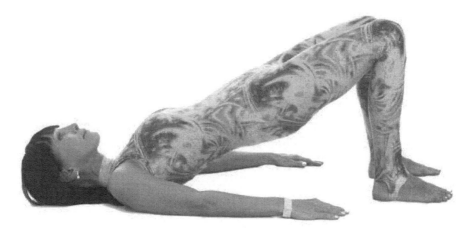

- At this point, your bodyweight is evenly distributed, and your hips level. Your aim during this pose is to **keep your hips level**. It is also very important that both your thighs also remain parallel throughout the pose – don't allow one thigh to rise higher than the other.

- Breathe in, and as you breathe out lift your right foot and extend your leg – remember to keep your thighs in line. Straight away you should feel that your right hip wants to drop – fight it! By trying to keep your hips straight and level you are using your core stability muscles very deeply. You may feel that familiar tremor as these muscles work!

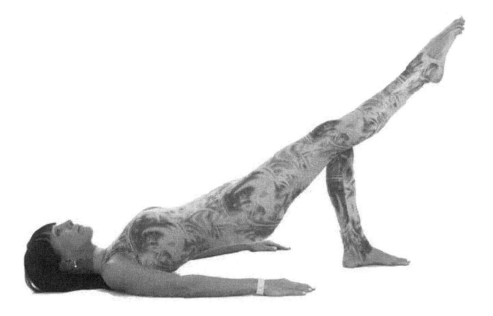

- Hold the pose for 3-5 deep breaths, and return your foot to the floor.

- Repeat with your left leg.

Note: You may feel your shoulders start to tense with the effort required for this pose. Try to keep your shoulders relaxed. Ensure your thighs remain level throughout the pose.

Mermaid Pose

Mermaid is a deceptively strong and effective workout for the torso – strengthening the Intercostal muscles and the Obliques, resulting in a stronger leaner torso and a smaller, tighter waist.

The Intercostal muscles are situated in between the ribs and are used to expand and contract the ribcage as we breathe. Mermaid is a particularly useful pose for those suffering from respiratory conditions where lung function is compromised, as strong Intercostal muscles will help the lungs to inflate fully, facilitating easier breathing. For this reason it is also a very good pose for sports people, especially runners, or simply if you get "puffed out" easily.

- Lie on your right-hand side with your body and legs in one straight line. Your right arm should be resting on the floor above your head, in line with your body and the palm of that hand facing the floor. Rest your head on your upper arm. Bend your left elbow and place the palm of your left hand on the floor in front of your chest with your elbow facing the ceiling. There should be a small gap between your body and your left hand.

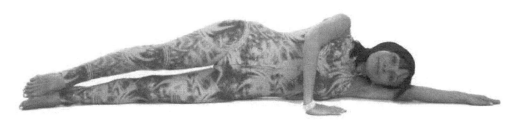

- Breathe in, and as you breathe out lift your upper body, and both legs, off the floor as high as you can. Keep both legs together, and lean slightly on your left arm for support.

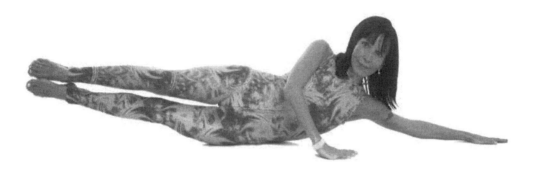

- Hold the pose for 5 deep breaths, and then relax to the floor. Repeat the pose twice more, and then roll over to your left-hand side and repeat from the start.

Note: Focus on keeping your legs together during this pose – the lift should come from the underneath leg, with your top leg simply acting as a weight. Keep both upper body and legs as high as possible – in this pose your body should resemble a curve shape.

When you are ready to work harder, you can add a small pulsing movement with your legs while holding your lift.

SECTION 4

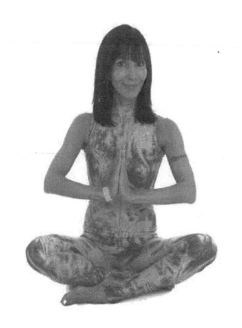

SPINAL POSES

SPINAL POSES

We have a poor record in the UK for back problems, and it is a sad fact that more work days are lost each year in this country because of back ailments than for any other reason.

Very often, the root cause of a back problem is simply weak spinal muscles, which in turn affects the posture and skeletal system, resulting in damage to the spine and surrounding musculature. It makes sense, then, to strengthen the muscles of the back, so that they support the skeletal system properly, thus improving posture, and consequently significantly reducing the likelihood of back problems.

It is also vital that we stretch our spinal muscles regularly. We all suffer from a certain amount of spinal compression. We cannot avoid this - it is because we are upright on two legs. Gravity is bearing down on us constantly, regardless of whether we are standing or sitting, and over a period of time this can cause the vertebrae to become compacted. In turn this can have an adverse impact on the delicate discs in between our vertebrae. By stretching the spinal muscles as described in this section, you can significantly reduce the risk of developing a problem like a prolapsed (slipped) disc or a trapped nerve condition such as Sciatica.

Cat Pose

This great pose stretches and tones the spinal muscles, and gently loosens up the back, reducing backache, eliminating stiffness and restoring suppleness. While its primary function is to strengthen and mobilise the spine, it will also tone the abdominal muscles

- **Cat Pose** is performed on hands and knees. You should ensure your knees are well protected, by kneeling on a cushion or folded towel. Your hands should be placed on the floor directly underneath your shoulders, arms straight and fingers facing forward, and your knees should be directly underneath each hip. Keep your spine relaxed and in a neutral position.

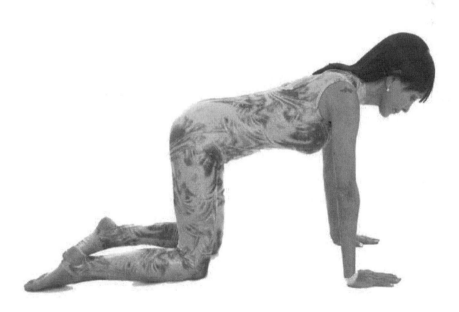

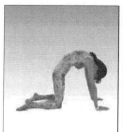 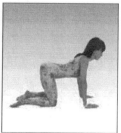

- Take a deep breath in, and as you breathe out, lift and round your spine up towards the ceiling, pulling your abdominal muscles in, pushing your hips forward (tucking your tailbone under), and allow your head to drop down. This movement should be done slowly and smoothly, in conjunction with your breath **out**.

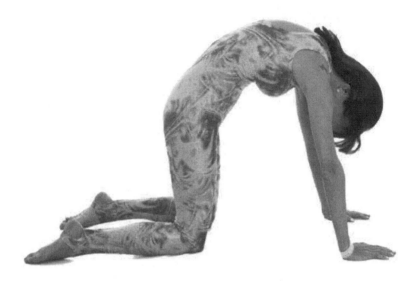

- Once you have completed your breath out, hold this position for approximately thirty seconds. During this time breathe gently, keeping your abdominal muscles pulled in and your back rounded. It is during this time that you are strengthening and toning your abdominals as well as stretching your spinal muscles.

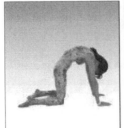 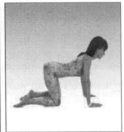

- Now, slowly breathe in as you "reverse" the movement – arch your spine, aiming your ribcage down towards the floor, pushing your bottom up towards the ceiling, and bring your head up **until it is in line with your spine** - do not tilt your head any further back. This movement should also be done slowly and smoothly, in conjunction with your breath **in.**

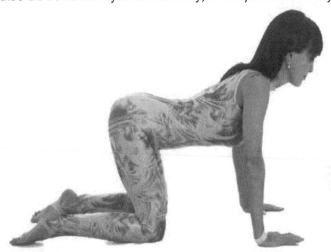

- Again, hold this position for approximately thirty seconds, breathing gently, before returning your spine to a neutral position.

- At this stage, you have now performed the two movements of **Cat Pose** and held each movement still for a short period. Now, to complete the pose, put the two movements together, in time with your breathing, allowing your spine to "flow" smoothly from one position to the other.

- These two movements should now be performed, in conjunction with your breathing and without stopping in between, until you have completed five of each.

Note: Take your time - these movements should be very slow and controlled. Remember to keep your breathing as slow and full as possible (i.e. filling your lungs completely as you breathe in and emptying them totally as you breathe out).

If you are unable to kneel, this posture can be done standing: Keeping your knees slightly bent, lean forward, arms outstretched, and position your hands against a wall, at the same height and width as your shoulders. Walk your hands down the wall until your torso is parallel with the floor. Ensure that your heels are underneath your hips and keep your knees slightly bent for the whole of the exercise.

Active Cat Pose

*Active Cat adds more movement to the traditional **Cat Pose**. By focussing on one side of the body at a time, **Active Cat** provides a deeper stretch for the spine. The shoulders and pectoral muscles also work hard in this pose. **Active Cat** should only be attempted once the traditional **Cat Pose** can be done comfortably.*

- **Active Cat Pose** is performed on the hands and knees. You should ensure your knees are well protected, by kneeling on a cushion or folded towel. Your hands should be placed on the floor directly underneath your shoulders, arms straight and fingers facing forward, and your knees should be directly underneath each hip. Keep your spine relaxed and in a neutral position.

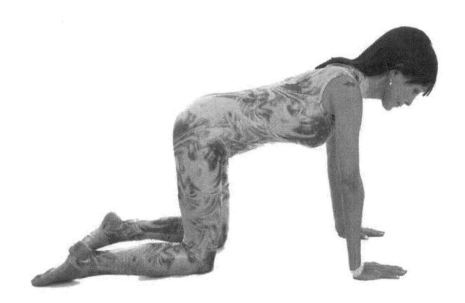

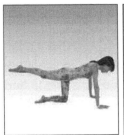 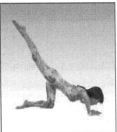 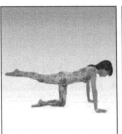 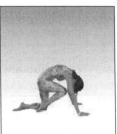

- On your first breath in, lift your right knee and extend your leg behind you, bringing it level with your body.

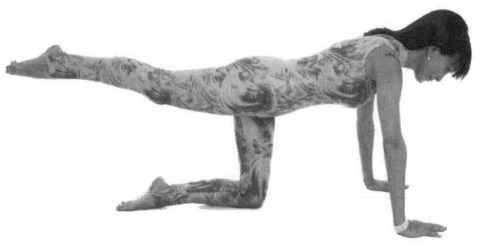

- As you breathe out, bend your elbows and lower your chest towards the floor (do not let it touch the floor). Your right leg should lift higher at the same time.

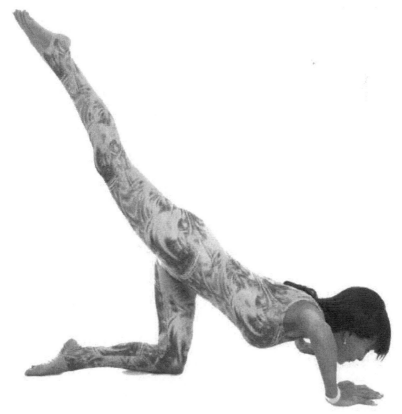

- On your next breath in straighten your arms and bring your right leg back in line with your body.

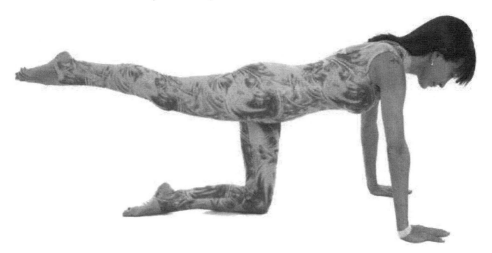

- Finally, on your next breath out your back rounds as you drop your head and bend your right knee in towards your head – try to bring your head and knee as close towards each other as possible.

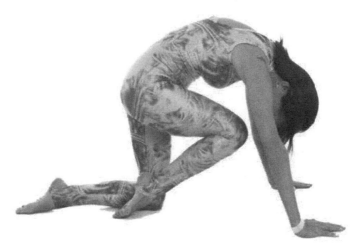

- Repeat 3 more times with your right leg, and return to your starting position.

- Repeat the above steps again, this time with your left leg extended.

Note: **The movements in Active Cat are done slowly, and should be synchronised with your breathing. For maximum effect, focus on getting both your breathing and movements slower each time you perform this pose.**

Spinal Realignment Pose

This pose has two primary functions – firstly, as the name suggests, it will realign and stretch your spine; secondly, it will strengthen your core stability muscles – the stabilising muscles of the abdomen and pelvis. This posture also requires a certain degree of balance, and this will teach you how to focus your mind, and improve your powers of concentration.

- Come onto your hands and knees. Ensure that your hands are directly underneath your shoulders with your fingers facing forward, and that your knees are directly underneath your hips. Keep your neck in line with the spine, by looking down at the floor.

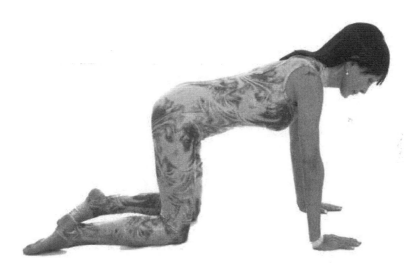

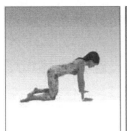 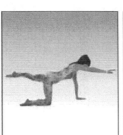 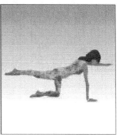

- Take a deep breath in, and as you breathe out raise your right arm straight up in front of you until it is level with your shoulder, palm facing down. Stretch your arm as though you were trying to touch something just beyond your reach. Take another deep breath in, and as you breathe out this time stretch your left leg out behind you, lifting it until it is level with the rest of your body. Again, imagine you are trying to touch something just beyond reach with your toes, and really feel the stretch in that leg!

- At this stage, your body should be in one straight line from the fingertips of your right hand, through to the toes of your left foot. You are likely to find yourself wobbling a little! Focus on your deep, slow breathing and try to get yourself in perfect balance, with both hips facing the floor, and hold the pose as still as possible.

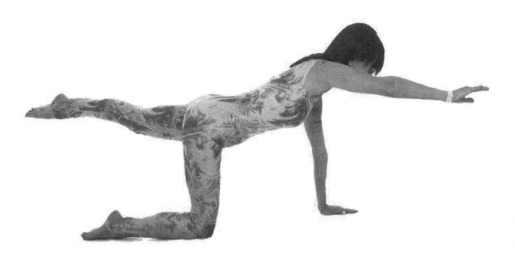

- Hold the pose for approximately 30 seconds, keeping your right arm and left leg perfectly level with your body. Then carefully return your arm and leg to your starting position.

- Now repeat the movement with your left arm and right leg. Remember to bring your arm into position first, before attempting to lift and stretch your leg out behind you. Again hold the pose for approximately 30 seconds, before returning your arm and leg to the floor.

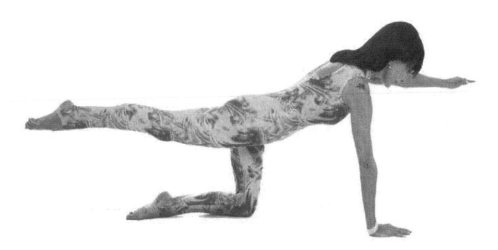

- You have now completed **Spinal Realignment Pose**. It is recommended that you now come into **Child Pose** for up to one minute, to allow your back and shoulder muscles to relax.

Note: In Spinal Realignment Pose, you may be tempted to tuck the toes of your foot on the floor, to help keep your balance. Try not to do this as it means you will be stabilising yourself with your foot. Instead, keep your toes untucked – and as a result your core stability muscles will be forced to work instead to keep you balanced. This will give you much better results.

Your goal with this pose is to maintain the position with no wobbling, and keep your body, from fingertips to toes, in one straight line. You may find this difficult at first, but with practice you will be surprised at how well you do - when your mind and body are in perfect harmony you will be able to hold this pose absolutely still!

Locust Pose

Locust is a very effective pose to strengthen the muscles of the lower back which, as a general rule, tends to be the most problematic area of the back. As an added bonus, it also tones and tightens the gluteal muscles, so your bottom will also be getting a workout!

- *Locust* is performed lying on your front. Rest on your forehead, so that your neck remains in alignment with your spine. Your arms should be straight down by your sides, with your fists clenched and resting on the floor, thumb-side down. Alternatively you may tuck your hands just underneath your hip bones, or simply press your palms firmly on the floor by your sides.

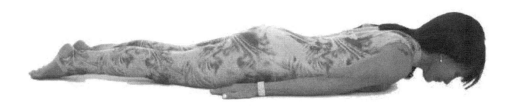

- Take a deep breath in, and as you breathe out, slowly lift your right leg just off the floor. Keep your leg straight, with your toes pointed. You do not need to lift your leg high – just aim to bring the front of your thigh an inch or two off the floor. Hold this position for 3 deep breaths, keeping your leg as stretched as possible. Then, slowly return your leg to the floor as you breathe out.

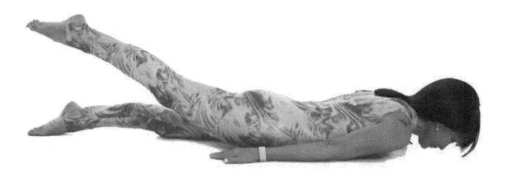

- Now repeat with your left leg.

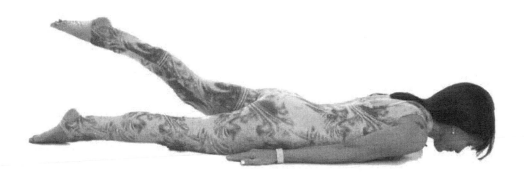

- Next, press the insides of your thighs, knees and feet firmly together, take a deep breath in, and as you breathe out lift **both** legs off the floor, keeping them as straight as possible. Try to keep the fronts of your thighs completely off the floor. Your legs **must** remain pressed together. Hold this stage of the pose for 5 deep breaths and then slowly return your legs to the floor.

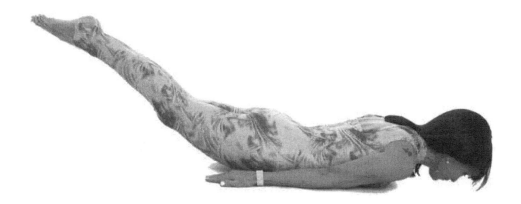

- Finally, repeat this stage again, but now also lift your upper body off the floor – lifting from the chest and **not** the neck. Raise and stretch your arms out behind you as though you were trying to touch your fingertips to your heels. Hold this stage of the pose for 5 deep breaths and then gently relax to the floor.

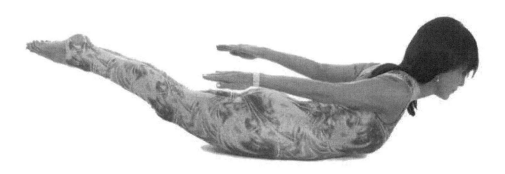

Note: During the latter two stages of Locust your legs will naturally want to separate, but you must try to keep them "glued" together. This requires considerable effort, so try not to tense your shoulders and neck.

During the final stage, make sure you do not tilt your neck back. Always aim to keep your neck in line with your spine.

Cobra Pose

Cobra, like **Locust**, is aimed at strengthening the lumbar spine muscles. It is a 3-stage pose – the first two stages being to strengthen the lower back muscles, and the third stage to improve flexibility in the spine. Over time your lower back muscles will strengthen considerably. Your shoulder and upper back muscles are also used to perform **Cobra** and will therefore become stronger, and in addition, your abdomen will become more toned if you breathe correctly during the final stage (pulling the abdominal muscles in, as you breathe out).

Stage 1
- **Cobra** is performed lying on your front. Rest on your forehead, so that your neck remains in alignment with your spine. Your arms should be straight and down by your sides, with your palms flat on the floor.

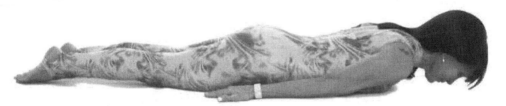

- Take a deep breath in, and as you breathe out slowly lift your head, shoulders and chest off the floor. Do not tilt your head back as you lift - your neck must remain in alignment with your spine at all times, to protect the delicate cervical vertebrae. Once you have lifted your upper body as high as you can comfortably manage, hold this position for 3-5 deep breaths. Make sure your legs and feet remain relaxed and on the floor.

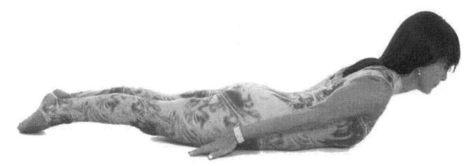

- When you have completed your deep breaths, allow your body to slowly return to the floor with your next breath out. Relax here for thirty seconds before going on to Stage 2.

Stage 2

- Now bend your elbows, bringing them in to the sides of your body, and tuck them in as close to your waist as you can manage. Your elbows, through to your fingertips, should be on the floor. Your arms must remain in this position during Stage 2.

- Breathe in, and as you breathe out once again lift your head, shoulders and chest off the floor as high as you can, (remember to keep your neck in line with your spine) and hold for 3-5 deep breaths. Fight the urge to let your elbows slide forward – if they do, your arms are then supporting you and your back muscles are not working!

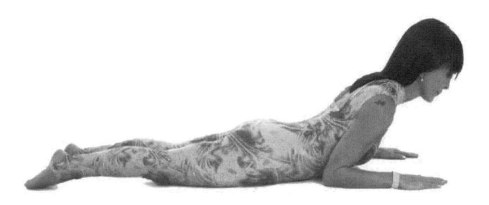

- When you have completed your deep breaths, allow your body to slowly return to the floor with your next breath out. Relax here for thirty seconds before going to Stage 3.

Stage 3

- Now, let your elbows lift and slide your hands forwards to just above shoulder level, and place them slightly wider than shoulder width. Your hands should be flat on the floor, with your fingers facing forward and your elbows pointed upward. Breathe in, and as you breathe out use your arms to push your upper body off the floor. Your arms should not straighten completely – keep a bend on your elbows – and your hips should remain on the floor. Relax your shoulders and lengthen your neck – aim to get as much distance between your shoulders and ear lobes as possible.

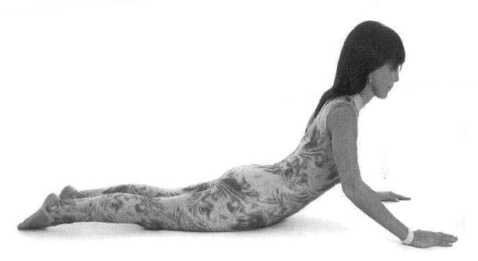

- This final stage completes the full **Cobra Pose**. The deep breathing is particularly important during this stage. Focus on lifting your chest and expanding your rib cage as much as you can each time you breathe in, taking full advantage of the fact that, in this position, you have created extra space in which your lungs can inflate completely. As you breathe out, pull your abdominal muscles in as much as you can to feel a wonderful stretch throughout the whole abdominal area. This stretch in itself is a great toning exercise for the abdominal muscles. Continue to breathe deeply, aiming for at least 5 deep breaths.

- After 5 deep breaths, push yourself back onto hands and knees. From here, drop your bottom to your heels and come into **Child Pose** to relax for one minute.

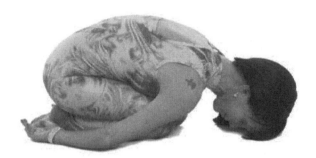

Note: During the first two stages of Cobra Pose, you will be aware of a "tight" feeling in your lower back, almost as though you are wearing a tight belt. This is the contraction of your lumbar spine muscles, working hard and growing stronger in the process. That tightness is telling you that you are doing a good job!

Take care not to tilt your head back as you lift your upper body off the floor in the first two stages. Focus on lifting your upper body from your chest, rather than from your neck. Keep your neck in line with your spine at all times during this pose.

Open (Partial) Bow Pose

Open – or Partial – Bow is a gentler version of Bow Pose. In Open Bow, all the muscles of the back are put to work and strengthened, along with the muscles of the shoulders, and the gluteal muscles too. This is a 3- tiered pose, gently building up to the final stage, giving you a safe and effective way to a strong and healthy spine.

- Lie on your front, resting on your forehead, with your arms outstretched and resting on the floor above your head, about one metre apart. Take your legs out behind you to about a one metre width, bringing you into a "jumping jack" shape.

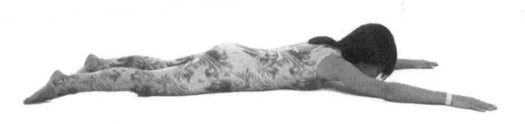

- Take a deep breath in, and as you breathe out lift your head, right arm and left leg off the floor. Your limbs should remain straight, and your neck must remain in line with your spine – do not tilt your head back. Hold this position for 3 deep breaths before gently returning to the floor.

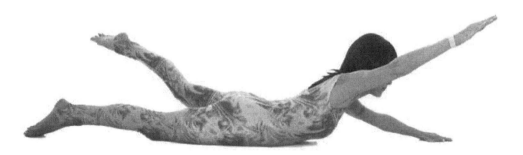

- Repeat with your left arm and right leg.

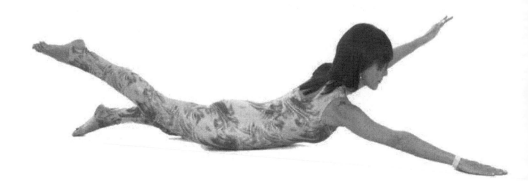

- Finally, breathe in and as you breathe out raise your head, both arms and both legs. Hold for 3 deep breaths and return to the floor. Repeat this final stage twice more.

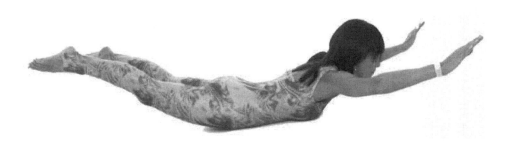

Note: It is important that you do not tilt your neck back when you lift your head. Focus on keeping your neck in line with your spine, lifting from your chest rather than your neck. Try to retain your "jumping jack" position in the final stage of the pose.

At this final stage, you are using – and strengthening – not only all your back muscles, but your shoulders, upper abdominal muscles, gluteal muscles and hamstrings too!

Bow Pose

This pose flexes the spine strongly, keeping the back mobile and flexible. I strongly recommend that you complete **Open Bow** *prior to attempting the full* **Bow Pose**, *so that your back muscles are warmed up and primed for this much harder pose.*

- Lie on your front, resting on your forehead, with your arms down by your side and your feet together on the floor behind you.

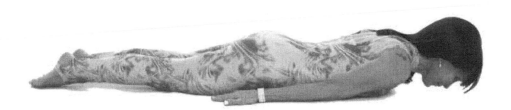

- Bend your knees, and bring your heels to your bottom. Reach back and take hold of each of your ankles with your hands.

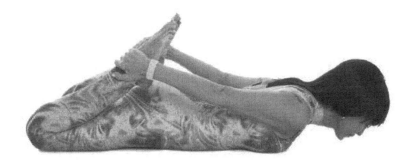

- Breathe in, and as you breathe out lift your upper body off the floor and raise your thighs, lifting your feet up toward the ceiling. You are aiming to create as much distance between your bottom and your heels as you can.

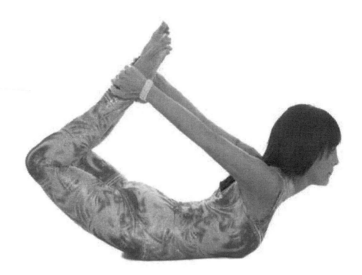

- Hold the pose for 3-5 deep breaths, and release to the floor.

Note: **This is a strong flexing pose for the spine, and therefore I now recommend that you come straight into Child Pose to counter-stretch your spine, allowing the muscles to relax. Simply place your hands on the floor either side of your shoulders, push yourself up onto your knees and drop straight into Child Pose from there. Relax here for 5 deep breaths.**

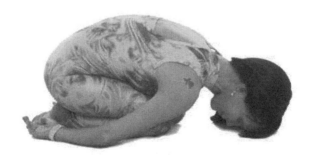

Forward Bend/Fan Pose

Forward Bend *strengthens the hips and stretches the hamstrings – back thigh muscles – an area known for being tight and under-stretched. If left unchecked, tight hamstrings can tug on the lower back muscles and pull them out of alignment, causing back ache. So, by regularly stretching the hamstrings you will be helping to avoid lower back problems.*

Also, well stretched hamstrings are much less vulnerable to injury – an important factor for runners and sportspeople.

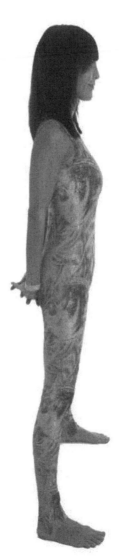

- Stand tall, with your feet approximately one metre apart. Your legs should be straight, with your toes facing forward. Draw back your shoulders, link your hands behind your back and rest your hands on your bottom. Your arms should be straight.

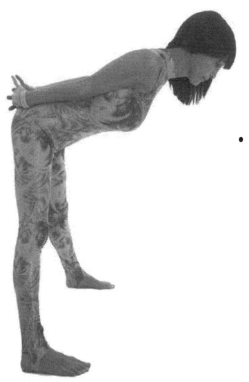

- Take a breath in and as you breathe out start to bend forwards from the hips, pressing your tailbone out behind you and leading down with your chest. Your head and neck stay in line with your spine. Stop when your torso is in a horizontal position. Finally, push your bodyweight from your heels over onto your toes. This may make you feel like you are about to topple forwards – this is a sign you are in the correct position.

- Hold your *Forward Bend* for 3-5 deep breaths.

Note: You will now feel a strong stretch at the back of your thighs and behind your knees. If this becomes too uncomfortable, allow both knees to bend slightly. Try to keep your back straight throughout the pose, by drawing your shoulders back and pressing your tailbone upwards continually.

Fan Pose

Fan Pose is performed as a continuation from **Forward Bend**. **Fan Pose** is a gentle stretch for the spine and shoulders. It will also tighten your waist and strengthen the Intercostal muscles. The Intercostal muscles are situated in between the ribs and are used to expand and contract the ribcage as we breathe. By strengthening these muscles, the expansion of the rib cage is increased, leading to improved lung function – making this an important pose for those suffering from respiratory conditions where lung function is compromised. It's also a great pose for the sports people amongst us, especially runners.

From **Forward Bend:**

- Release your hands, and place them on the floor directly underneath your shoulders. Keep your back straight, with your shoulders back and tailbone pressed upwards.

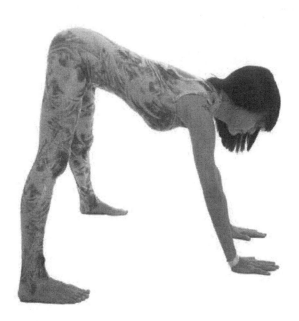

- Lift your right hand off the floor, and place it palm-side down onto your tailbone.

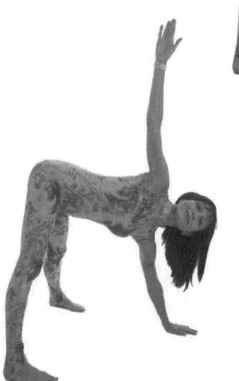

- Turn from your waist to your right-hand side, drawing your right shoulder as far back as possible. At the same time, bring your left shoulder as far forward as possible, to ensure maximum rotation in your torso. Now, stretch your right arm high, with the palm of your hand facing forwards.

- Hold for 3-5 deep breaths, then replace your right hand on the floor and repeat the pose with your left arm and turning to the left.

- To come out of Fan Pose, simply replace your left hand on the floor, bend your knees slightly and uncurl slowly from the base of your spine, to standing.

Note: Try to keep both legs straight while you are in Fan Pose. If this becomes too uncomfortable, allow both knees to bend slightly.

Spinal Circles

This gentle circling pose is a great way to loosen up stiffness in the lumbar spine and can bring instant relief to lower backache.

- Lie on your back, and hug your knees to your chest, keeping your feet together. Your hands should be placed over each knee.

- Start to "draw" small circles with your knees, both knees circling together and in the same direction. Aim to keep your circles as close to your body as possible, so gently pull your knees towards your body as you complete your circles.

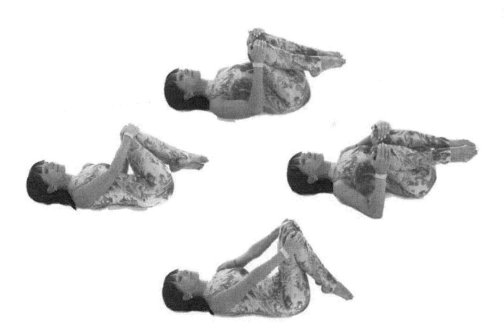

- "Draw" 5-8 circles in one direction, and repeat in the other direction.

Note: This pose will gently "massage" your lower back against the floor, easing away any tension in this area.

Converse Circles (Hip Circles)

This form of circling will loosen up stiffness in the hips and can help to increase range of movement in the hip area too.

- Lie on your back, and hug your knees to your chest, keeping your feet together. Your hands should be placed over each knee.

- Start to "draw" circles with your knees – this time both knees circling in the opposite direction to each other. Keep the circles wide, and make sure you complete each circle by bringing the knees in together.

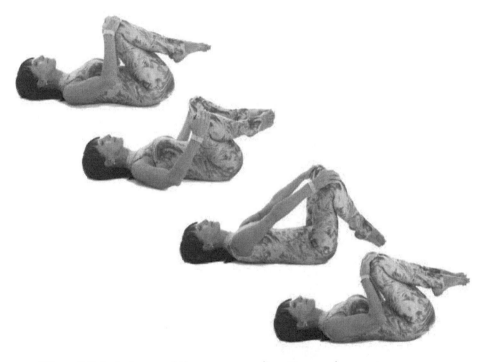

- "Draw" 5-8 circles, and then reverse direction and repeat.

Note: The hip is a "ball and socket" type joint. The movement involved in converse circling will rotate the head (the "ball") of your femur (thigh bone) in the socket of the hip, which is a very beneficial movement for mobility of the hips. This movement will also stimulate the production of synovial fluid, keeping the hip joints well lubricated.

Spinal Roll

A quick way to relieve a niggly backache, stretch your spine and stimulate blood flow to the spinal area.

- Lie on your back, and hug your knees to your chest, keeping your feet together. Start to roll back and forth along the length of your spine, using momentum to eventually propel yourself into a sitting position. Try to do at least 5 spinal rolls before you reach the seated finale!

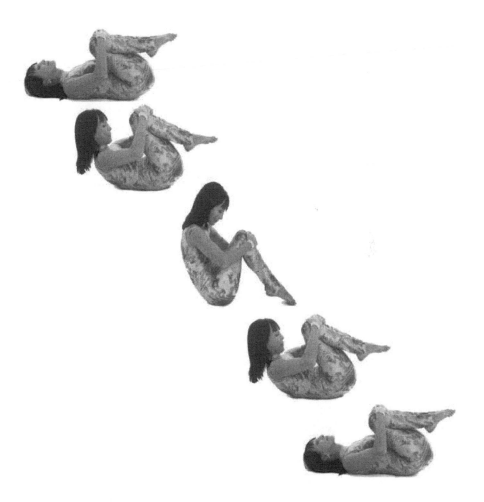

Note: This simple pose can work wonders if your back feels tired – for instance if you have been standing – or sitting - for a long period of time.

Supine Spinal Twist

This is a wonderful, gentle stretch for the spine, performed whilst lying on your back. It is relaxing and requires little effort, yet has some very important benefits:-

As we are standing or sitting for most of our time, gravity takes its toll and by the end of day the spine can become quite compressed, resulting in pain and stiffness. This pose very gently eases the vertebrae apart, reducing the pressure on the discs in between each vertebra. This not only helps to alleviate any stiffness, it also goes a long way to help prevent trapped nerves in your spine – for instance Sciatica - and prolapsed (slipped) discs.

*Your spine should be able to make 6 fundamental movements: a forward and backward bend, a side-to-side bend, and a side-to-side rotation. In **Supine Spinal Twist** your spine is rotated, and this will help to keep your spine fully mobile – it is the rotation function we tend to have difficulty with as we get older.*

***Supine Spinal Twist** also gently stretches and strengthens the spinal muscles, and improves posture.*

- Lie down on the floor on your back. Your knees should be bent, with the soles of your feet flat on the floor. Your knees and feet should be together, with your heels drawn quite close to your bottom. Bring your arms out to each side, level with your shoulders, and in a "T" shape with your body. Keep your arms straight and let them rest on the floor, with the palms of your hands facing down.

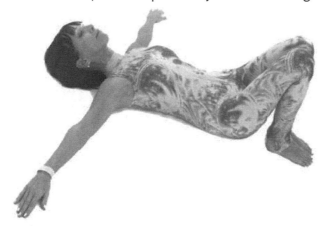

- Take a deep breath in, and as you slowly breathe out, let both legs drop over to your right hand side – gently "push" them over from your left hip. Try to keep both knees and feet on top of each other. Once your legs have rested into this position, turn your head to face your left-hand side. You should feel that your lower back has left the floor, and your left shoulder may have lifted a little as well. Close your eyes, and focus on your breathing, taking in long, slow, full breaths as you inhale, and making sure you exhale completely as well. Try to relax and enjoy the stretch!

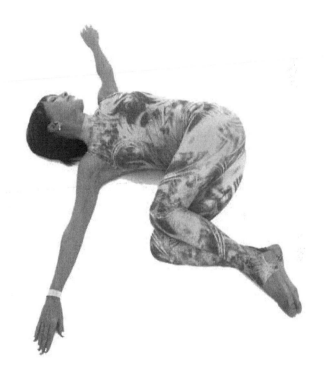

- You should be aware of a gentle pulling sensation in your spine as the vertebrae are being rotated and eased apart, releasing the pressure on the discs. The spinal muscles are also being stretched, and if you are breathing deeply you are allowing the whole area to be suffused with a good supply of oxygenated blood, feeding and nourishing the spine and surrounding muscles. The turning of your neck in the opposite direction to your legs ensures that your neck (cervical) vertebrae are also benefiting from the stretch.

- Stay in this position for approximately 2 minutes, and then breathe in as you bring your legs back into their starting position (the knees should still be bent, feet on the floor). Your head also turns back to its starting position.

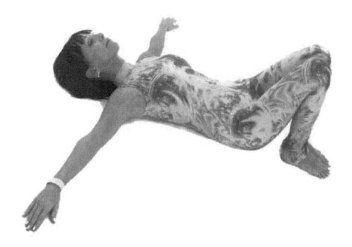

- On your next breath out, allow both legs to drop to your left-hand side, again gently "pushing" from your right hip, and trying to keep your knees together. When your legs are in place, turn your head to face your right-hand side. Once again, focus on your breathing, and relax your body.

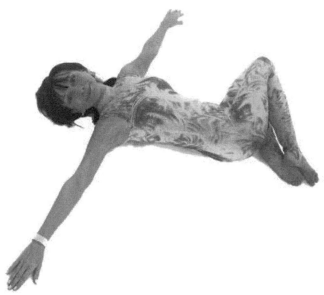

- Stay in this position for approximately 2 minutes, and then slowly breathe in as you return your knees and head to their starting position.

- Complete the pose by hugging both knees to your chest, lengthening the spine, and rocking gently from side to side – just an inch either side of the spine – for 30 seconds or so.

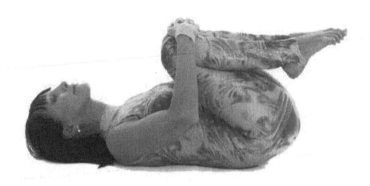

Note: If practiced daily, Supine Spinal Twist will help to keep your spine mobile and supple, decompressing the vertebrae, releasing pressure on the discs and stretching the spinal muscles. When performing Supine Spinal Twist, do not allow your feet to lift completely off the floor, which is commonly seen in this pose, as this can over-work your lower back muscles. By keeping your feet on the floor and allowing them to simply "peel" off the floor as you go from side to side, you have more control over the movement, making it safer.

Standing Cat Pose

This lovely little pose stretches the spine, shoulders and upper arms. It takes just seconds to perform, and can be done anywhere at any time of the day. A great pose to eliminate a niggly non-specific back-ache.

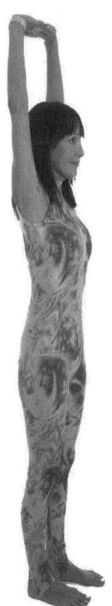

- Stand tall, with your feet a few inches apart, toes turned forward. As you breathe in raise both arms high and interlace your fingers, turning your palms up towards the ceiling. As you breathe out, stretch your arms as high as you can.

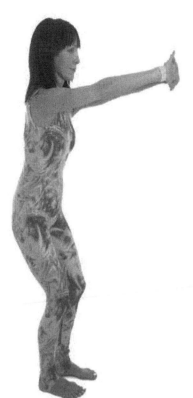

- Maintaining this stretch, bring your arms down in front of you until they are at shoulder level with the backs of your hands at eye level. Slightly bend your knees. Continue to pull your hands as far away from you as possible – your back should be well rounded at this stage.

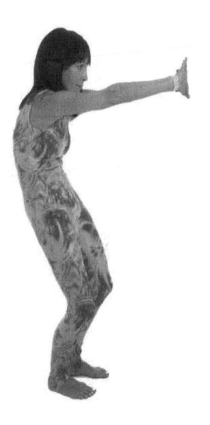

- Bend your knees more, and perform a deep pelvic tilt – imagine you are trying to point your lower abdominal area to the ceiling.

- You should now be feeling a strong stretch across your shoulders and running down the length of your spine. Hold this stretch for 3-5 deep breaths and release.

Note: This gentle but effective stretch can temporarily decompress the spine and relieve back-ache. The upper body stretch and the pelvic tilt must be maintained as strongly as possible throughout the pose.

SECTION 5

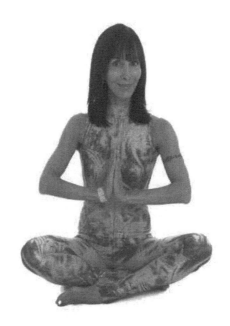

ABDOMINAL POSES

The abdominal area of the body, for most people, tends to be where the muscles are weakest – and yet this where we most need our muscles to be strong. Strong abdominal muscles will support the core area of the body, helping to prevent back problems and keeping body alignment – posture – correct. Weak abdominal muscles often go hand-in-hand with back problems, as the back muscles have to over-work to support the core area, putting them under strain.

It makes sense, then, to keep the abdominal muscles strong and firm – and apart from the fact that strong abdominals will do their job of supporting the core area of the body much more efficiently, from an aesthetic viewpoint a "washboard stomach" or "six-pack" is on most people's wish list!

There's no doubt that while the poses in this section are tough, they WILL give you results if you bear with them and be patient.

Abdominal Hollowing

*This pose gives you a gentle but effective workout for the abdominal muscles. By contracting the abdominal muscles against the resistance of gravitational pull, you are building up core strength, tightening and toning the abdominal area. With **Abdominal Hollowing,** there is no stress whatsoever placed on the spine, making this the perfect pose for anyone with a back problem. With regular practice, this pose will strengthen the abdominal muscles, enabling them to support the core area more effectively. With improved core support from the abdominal muscles, many back problems can be greatly improved.*

- Stand with your feet hip-width apart, toes turned forward. Slightly bend your knees and lean over, resting your hands on your thighs, with your fingers turned inward. (Do not rest your hands on your knees.) Let your elbows bend slightly out to each side.

  Allow your bodyweight to rest on your arms, so that your back is comfortable. Your back should be gently rounded, so tuck your tailbone under, and let your head drop.

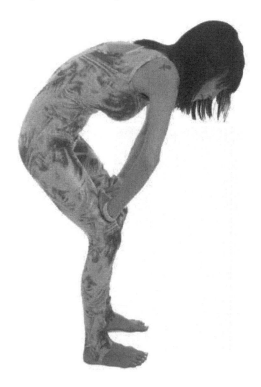

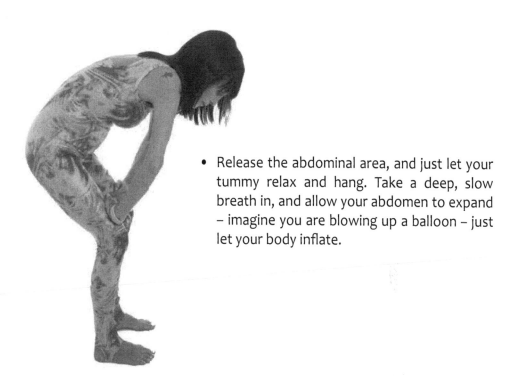

- Release the abdominal area, and just let your tummy relax and hang. Take a deep, slow breath in, and allow your abdomen to expand – imagine you are blowing up a balloon – just let your body inflate.

- As you breathe out slowly, draw your abdominal muscles inward and upward – as though you were trying to touch your navel to your spine. You are trying to create a "hollow" in the abdominal area.

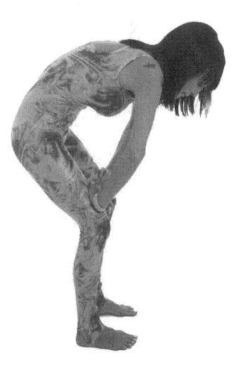

149

- Continue these two movements in line with your breathing, keeping them slow and controlled. Aim to complete a minimum of ten hollows before gently uncurling.

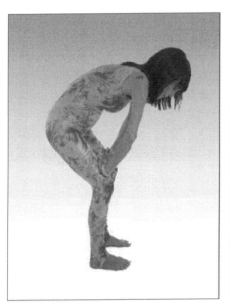 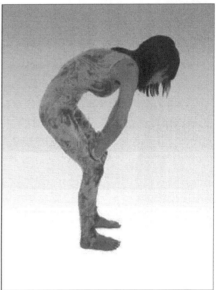

Note: Ensure that your fingers face inward (with elbows bending outward) during Abdominal Hollowing, as this minimises any stress on your wrists. However, if you have a pre-existing wrist problem and this begins to feel uncomfortable for your wrists, just drop a little lower with your body and rest on your forearms/elbows instead of on your hands.

The best time of day to do Abdominal Hollowing is first thing in the morning, straight out of bed – your stomach is empty, and your muscles have been relaxing overnight making them more compliant. They will work much harder for you!

Boat Pose

*I believe **Boat Pose** is the ultimate pose for the abdominal muscles – strengthening and toning not only the abdominals, but also the core stability muscles and the obliques (waist muscles). It involves a prolonged contraction, where the muscles remain contracted and held still for a period of time. It IS, undoubtedly, hard work so build up slowly, holding the pose for a very short time initially. With regular practice you will see the results of your hard work.*

- Lie on your back, with your knees bent and feet on the floor.

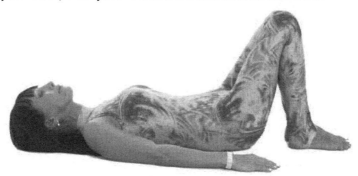

- Take a breath in, and as you breathe out, curl your upper body off the floor, and take hold around the outside of your thighs, as close to underneath your knees as you can reach. You should now be resting on your lower back, with everything above waist level off the floor. Keep your back and shoulders rounded.

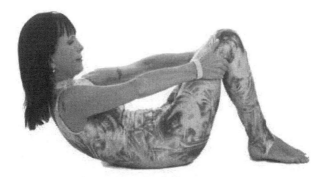

- Look down at your tummy, and next time you breathe out draw your abdominal muscles down towards the floor. Hold them firm and tight, whilst breathing normally.

- Lift your right foot off the floor, and raise it up until your leg is almost straight. Your right thigh remains level with your left thigh. Repeat with your left leg, which should leave you balancing just on your lower back.

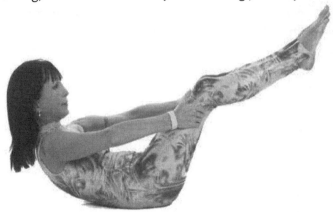

- Release your legs, and stretch your arms straight out in front of you. Draw your shoulders back, and bring your hands down until they are just a few inches above the floor.

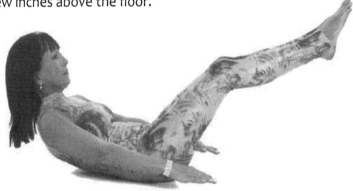

- You are now in **Boat Pose**. Hold the pose initially for 3 deep breaths, building up as you grow stronger, to a maximum of 20 breaths.

- When you are ready, release the pose gently, returning your head and both feet to the floor. Gently roll your head from side to side, to release any tension that may have built up in your neck.

Note: If you find your neck starts to ache during this pose, place one hand behind your head and allow the weight of your head to rest in your hand. Make sure that you keep your feet above knee level throughout the pose, to avoid placing stress on your lumbar spine.

Rocking Boat Pose

*A variation on **Boat Pose**, **Rocking Boat** introduces a gentle rocking movement, making the muscles work even harder. This pose should not be attempted until you are comfortable with the basic **Boat Pose**.*

- Lie on your back, with your knees bent and feet on the floor.

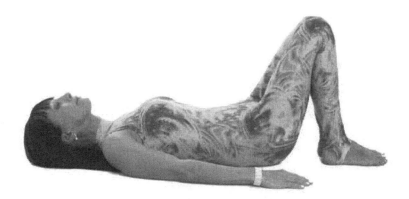

- Breathe in, and as you breathe out, curl your upper body off the floor, and take hold around the outside of your thighs, as close to underneath your knees as you can reach. You should now be on your lower back, with everything above waist level off the floor. Keep your back and shoulders rounded.

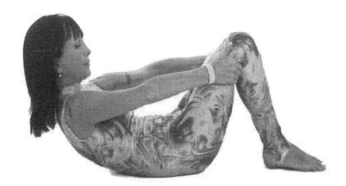

- Look down at your tummy, and next time you breathe out draw your abdominal muscles down towards the floor. Hold them firm and tight, whilst breathing normally.

- Lift both feet off the floor and bring your legs out into a diagonal position, with your feet above knee level. Cross your ankles.

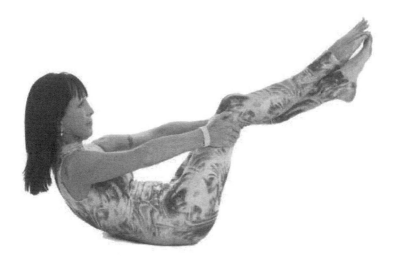

- Release your legs, and come into **Prayer Pose**, with your fingertips facing the ceiling.

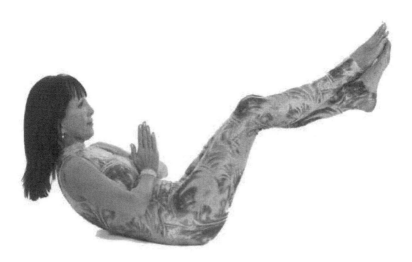

- Start to gently rock back and forth, over your lower back only. As your head comes up a few inches your feet should go down, and vice-versa. This is a relatively small movement, and should be done slowly. Breathe out as your head comes up, and breathe in on the way back.

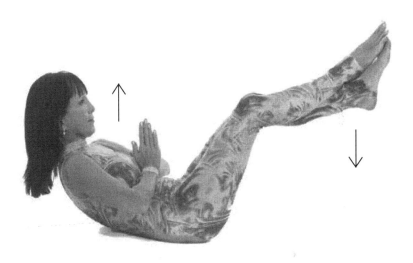

- Aim for 3-5 rocks. This can be increased at your own pace, as you become stronger.

Note: While rocking, try not to let your upper back touch the floor. You should rock over your lower back only. If you feel discomfort in your neck, place one hand behind your head.

If you find Rocking Boat difficult, start by holding on around your thighs . . . in time, as your abdominals grow stronger, you will be able to let go.

Extended Leg Pose

This is another very effective abdominal pose involving a prolonged contraction. **Extended Leg Pose** *will strengthen and tone your abdominal muscles, with the added bonus of strengthening the shoulders and stretching the hamstrings.*

- Lie on your back, with your knees bent. As you breathe out, raise your left leg straight up, flexing your foot so that the sole of your foot is facing the ceiling.

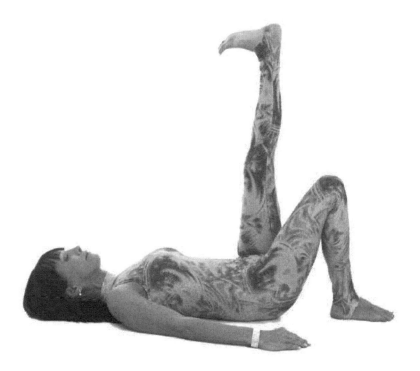

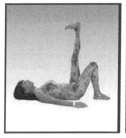 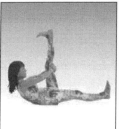 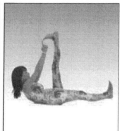

- Take hold behind your left thigh with both hands, and on your next breath out raise your upper body off the floor as high as you can manage. Now stretch your right leg straight out, just one inch off the floor, and flex your foot. At this point, both legs should be as straight as possible, and both feet flexed.

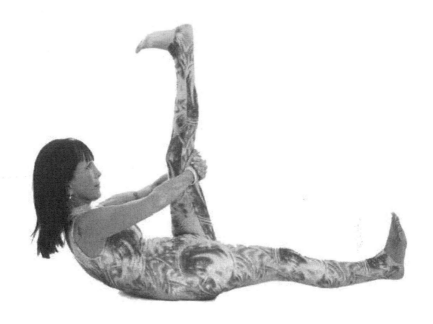

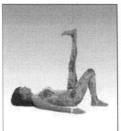 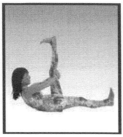 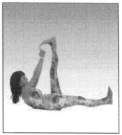

- Release your leg, and bring your hands into **Temple Pose**, with your index fingertips facing the ceiling. Start to raise your hands up towards your toes. At the same time, draw your toes down towards your fingertips – your aim is to continually try to close the gap between your toes and fingertips. If you are able to touch the two together, focus on maintaining that contact. Hold the pose for 3-5 deep breaths, and release to the floor.

- Repeat with your right leg raised.

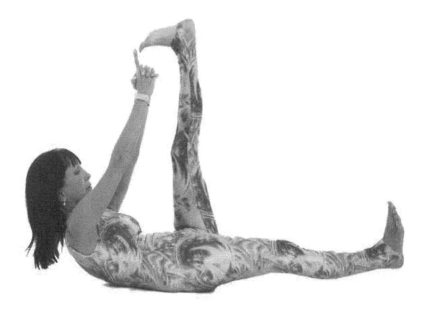

Note: If you find your neck starts to ache during this pose, place one hand behind your head and allow the weight of your head to rest in your hand. Simply stretch up towards your toes with just the other hand.

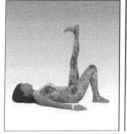 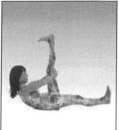 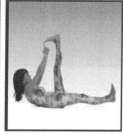

Split Bamboo Pose

Split Bamboo *is another fabulous pose to strengthen the abdominal area – this time focussing on* *transversus abdominis,* *the lower abdominals. This area of the abdominals tends to be the weakest part, and because of this, your lower back muscles may try to join in, to help your lower abdominals cope with the workload placed on them in this pose. You will know if this is happening – your lower back will start to arch. So, during this pose, your main focus must be on* *not allowing your back to arch. In Split Bamboo,* *we simply use the weight of the legs to strengthen the abdominals.*

- Lie on your back, with your knees bent and feet flat on the floor. Your arms rest on the floor by your sides. As you breathe out press down firmly with your abdominal muscles and try to "glue" your lower back onto the floor. You must now keep your abdominal muscles working continually, so that your lower back remains firmly pressed against the floor.

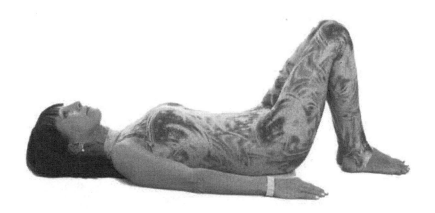

- Lift both legs up into the air, knees slightly bent.

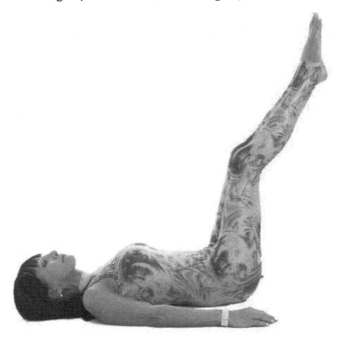

- Slowly start to lower down your right leg, until it is about half-way between your left leg and the floor.

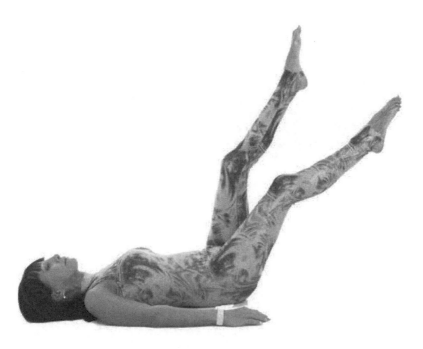

- Continually pressing down with your abdominal muscles to prevent your lower back arching, now start to lower down your left leg, but not as low as your right leg. Your left foot should remain just above your right foot.

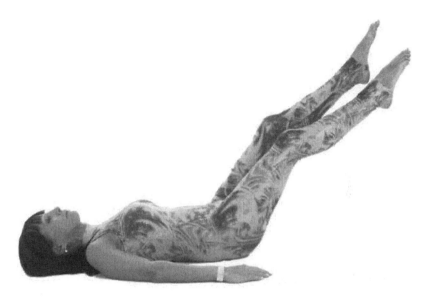

- At this stage you will find that your lower back is desperately trying to arch off the floor, to help your abdominals. Keep pressing down with your abdominals. Try to hold your pose for a slow count of 5 and then relax, allowing both knees to bend, and return your feet to the floor.

- Repeat the pose, with your left leg coming down first.

Note: In Split Bamboo Pose, you must continually contract your abdominals by pressing them firmly downwards, to the floor. If you feel your back beginning to arch, lift both legs a little higher and try to press down with your abdominal muscles again, to remove the arch in your spine. If your back continues to arch, release the pose immediately and relax. Focus on strengthening your abdominals with the other poses in this section – you can always attempt Split Bamboo Pose at a later date when your abdominals are a little stronger.

Make sure you don't hold your breath during the pose!

Scissor Pose

Scissor Pose *is a slow, graceful pose which should look as though it is being performed in slow motion. Its benefits are two-fold: it will strengthen and tone the abdominals, and it will also mobilise the hips, easing stiffness and improving mobility. The two movements should be performed slowly and precisely, and simultaneously with your breathing.*

- Lie on your back, with your knees bent and your feet flat on the floor.

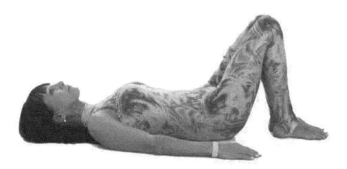

- Breathe in, and as you breathe out raise your right leg high into the air, pointing your toes to the ceiling.

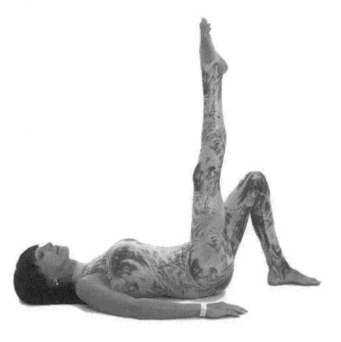

- Take hold behind your thigh with both hands and on your next breath out raise your upper body off the floor, bringing your chest towards your thigh. Stretch your left leg straight out in front of you, just one inch off the floor, and your toes pointed.

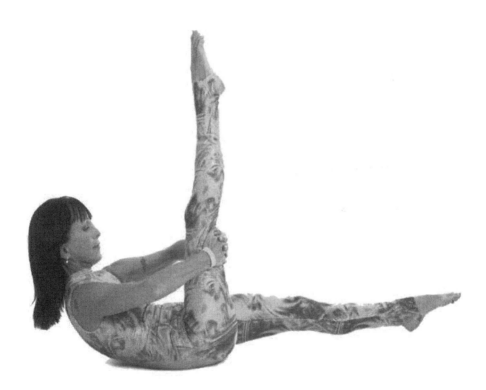

- As you breathe in, release your right leg and, without dropping your body, slowly change legs – raising your left leg and dropping your right leg down to one inch off the floor. Take hold behind your left thigh now, and as you breathe out curl your chest an inch closer towards your thigh.

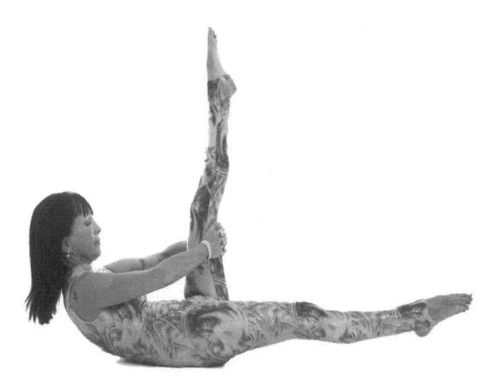

- Continue these two movements slowly, keeping both legs straight. Synchronise your movements with your breathing, making sure that you **change legs as you breathe in, and curl your chest closer to your thigh as you breathe out.**

- Aim for 8-10 sets – a set being both inhale and exhale.

Note: **Remember, this pose should be performed as though in slow motion. During the leg movements, try to keep your legs straight so that the movement comes from your hips and not your knees. As the name of this pose suggests, your legs should mimic scissors and remain as straight as possible.**

Plank Pose

Plank is a multi-faceted pose – it strengthens the abdominals, the muscles of the lower back and also the core stability muscles. Consequently it is a pretty tough pose! It's also a great shoulder strengthener.

- Lie on your front, propped up on your elbows. Your elbows should be placed directly under your shoulders, and your fingers linked together so that you have created a triangle shape with your forearms. Your legs should be straight out behind you, and together.

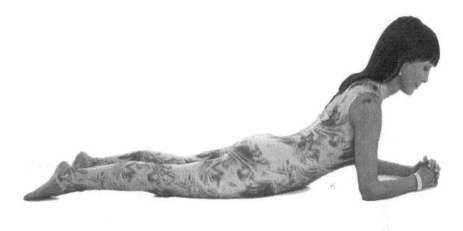

- Tuck your toes and bend your knees slightly, lifting your hips and the fronts of your thighs just off the floor. Your knees remain on the floor.

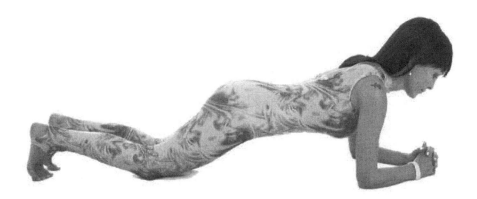

- Now straighten your legs, which will lift your knees off the floor. Adjust your body so that you are in a straight line from your head to your heels. Keep your abdominals pulled in and do not drop your head.

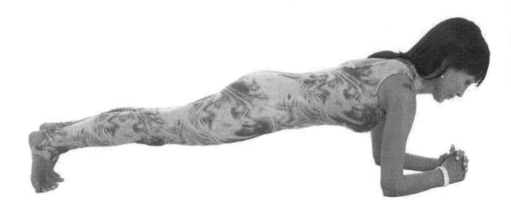

- Hold the pose for 5-8 deep breaths – increasing this as you become stronger.

- When you are ready, release the pose by returning your knees to the floor first.

Note: It is very easy to arch your back during Plank Pose and you must try to avoid this. Focus on keeping your tailbone tucked under, and continually lift from your shoulders to avoid "sinking" into your chest. If you feel discomfort in your lower back during Plank Pose, try lifting your bottom a little higher. If the discomfort persists, bend your knees back to the floor and relax immediately. Focus on strengthening your abdominals with the other poses in this section – you can always attempt Plank Pose at a later date when your abdominals are a little stronger.

SECTION 6

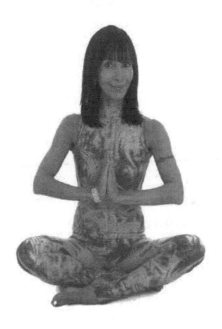

FLEXIBILITY POSES

FLEXIBILITY POSES

That old adage "If you don't use it, you lose it" is never more true than when it comes to flexibility! The way to a flexible body is by stretching the muscles regularly and consistently, and exercising the joints, tendons and ligaments. A more flexible, supple body is one of the main benefits of Hatha Yoga. Increased flexibility will improve your posture, which will help to prevent spinal and joint problems. Hatha Yoga stretches will lengthen the muscles, resulting in a longer, leaner more streamlined look to the body. A stretched muscle is a healthy muscle!

The secret to any stretch is to RELAX. Tension will always fight a stretch, so the more relaxed you can be, the better. Learn to release tension with your breath out. Visualise tension leaving your body with every breath out - like steam leaving a kettle. Let it go! Never force a stretch – always go just as far as you can comfortably manage, and then relax there.

One more important point: Don't expect an instant improvement in your flexibility. It takes time, but as long as you are patient and consistent with your practice, you WILL become more flexible. DO NOT OVER-STRETCH. Listen to what your body is telling you – while you should feel the stretch, you should NOT feel pain. Always take your time.

Butterfly Pose

This pose has many benefits, including:

- *Stretching and strengthening the spinal muscles and ligaments*
- *Removing tension from the neck and shoulders*
- *Toning the adductor (inner thigh) muscles*
- *Improving the posture and blood flow to the lower body*

Butterfly Pose *can also help to prevent sagging of the upper body and rounded shoulders. In time you will also find that your thighs become firmer, and your spine more flexible.*

- **Butterfly Pose** is performed sitting on the floor. Bend your knees and bring the soles of your feet together. Take your heels as close as possible to your groin, and hold around your toes with both hands. Without letting go of your feet, let your knees drop out to each side. Try and sit as tall as you can, with your neck long, your shoulders drawn back and your spine straight.

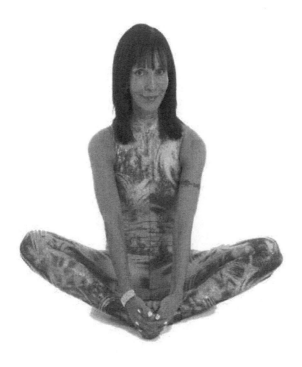

- Take a deep, slow breath in, and as you do so, round your back and drop your head down, and bring your knees right up to touch the sides of your arms. In effect, you are trying to curl yourself into a small tight ball.

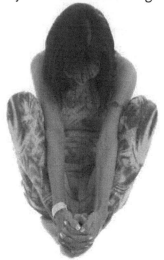

- Breathe out, and as you do so, straighten and stretch your spine, lengthen your neck, draw your shoulders back and push your knees down towards the floor – imagine you are trying to get your knees to touch the floor.

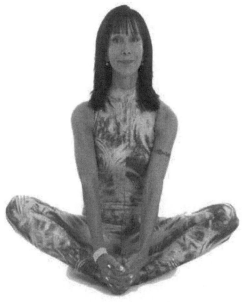

- Continue to repeat these two movements, slowly and smoothly, and synchronising each movement with your breathing, until you have done ten of each.

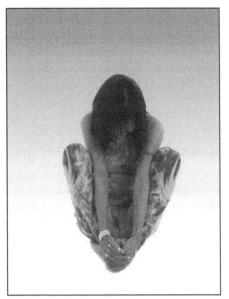 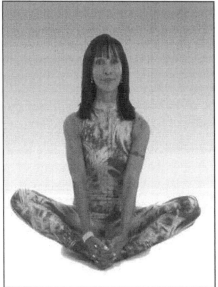

Note: Butterfly Pose consists of two main movements, both of which are performed in conjunction with your breathing. It is vital, therefore, to focus on breathing slowly and deeply, matching each movement to the breath, allowing the movements to flow freely from one to the other.

As you perform Butterfly Pose, think about perfecting your technique – curl yourself into an even smaller ball each time you breathe in, and with each breath out stretch your back a little more, pushing your knees even closer to the floor. You should really be aware of your muscles working as you perform these movements.

Diamond Pose

Diamond Pose *is a stretch for the lower body and will loosen stiff hips, stretch the lower back, and boost the blood supply to the area, leading to increased flexibility and suppleness of the spine. It will also tone the thighs and help to alleviate Sciatica.*

- Sit on the floor, with your legs stretched out in front of you. Bring the soles of your feet together – your knees should naturally bend out to each side as you do this. Slide your feet as far away from you as possible while keeping the soles of your feet together, so you have created a long "diamond" shape with your legs.

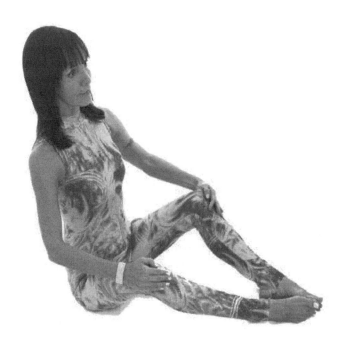

- Sit up as tall as you can, lengthening your spine and neck, with your hands resting on your knees.

- Take a deep breath in, and as you breathe out, slowly slide your hands down your shins towards your ankles, letting your chest ease down towards the floor in front of you. Take hold of your feet, resting your elbows outside your shins. Allow your body to relax, and let your head gently drop down. Breathe slowly and deeply, and focus on letting any tension leave your body as you breathe out. You should feel this stretch in your lower back, hips and thighs. Take two deep breaths here.

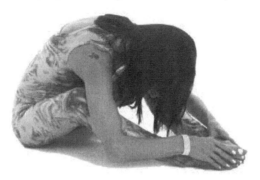

- Now, still holding your feet, lift your elbows, bring them inside your legs and drop them down toward the floor. Release your feet, draw your elbows in towards you, slide your hands underneath your ankles and wrap your hands around your feet.

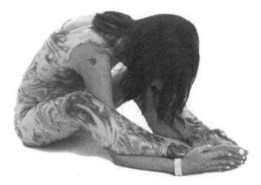

- Stay in this pose for one to two minutes, focussing on relaxing a little more with every breath out. The less tension in your body, the better you will stretch.

Note: **Don't worry if you cannot manage the final stage – just hold on to wherever you can comfortably reach, your shins for example, and relax over your legs. Your body will become more flexible over time with this stretch, and gradually you will get closer to your feet!**

3-stage Jack-knife Pose (Seated Forward Fold)

*This is a fabulous stretch, focussing on the lower back, hips and hamstrings - areas of the body notorious for being tight and stiff. **3-stage Jack-knife** will improve flexibility and mobility in the spine and hips, and significantly reduce hamstring injuries – so, a great pose for sportsmen/women!*

Stage 1

- Sit on the floor with your legs stretched out in front of you. Your spine should be long and straight, and your head upright. Bend your left knee out to the side, take hold of your ankle and pull your foot towards you. Place the sole of your foot to the inside of your right thigh, and let your left knee drop as close to the floor as possible.

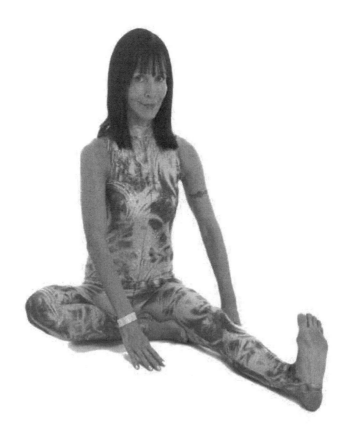

- Maintaining your long, straight spine, place your hands on the floor either side of your right leg. Your right foot should be flexed. Take a deep breath in, and as you breathe out "walk" your hands down towards your foot as far as you can manage comfortably. If you can reach your foot, hold on to your ankle or underneath your foot with both hands, to keep you "anchored" in position. Don't worry if you cannot reach your foot – just hold on to your shin instead, or keep your hands on the floor if you prefer. Try to relax into the pose, feeling the stretch, and hold it for 3-5 deep breaths before "walking" your hands back up.

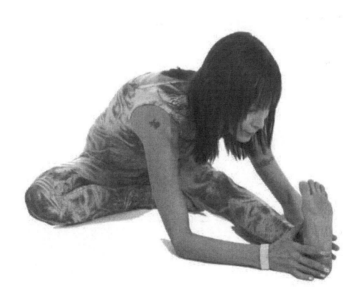

Stage 2

- Straighten out your left leg, and check to make sure your back is still tall and straight. Now repeat the steps of Stage 1, this time with your right knee bent, and stretching over your extended left leg.

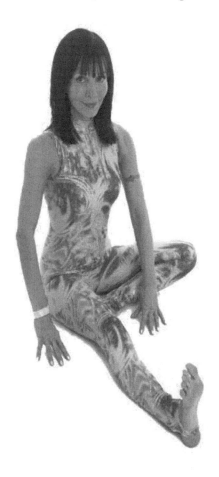

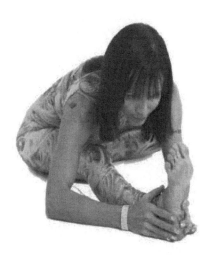

Stage 3

- Sit tall, with both legs straight out in front of you, and your feet flexed. Place your hands on the floor either side of your legs, take a deep breath in, and as you breathe out "walk" your hands down towards your feet, bringing your chest down towards your legs. Take hold of your shins/ankles/underneath your feet with both hands and just relax over your legs.

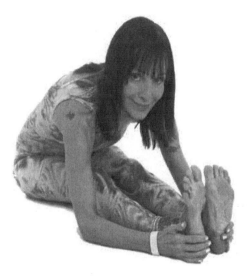

- Let the tension dissolve away with every breath out, and you will slowly feel yourself drop closer to your legs as your body relaxes. Hold the pose for 3-5 deep breaths.

Note: At each stage of this pose, aim to bring your chest down towards your thighs, so your back remains relatively straight, as opposed to rounding the spine and dropping your head down.

This pose brings on a strong stretch at each stage, and you will feel this in your lower back, hips, thighs and hamstrings. Focus on your deep breathing, and stay as relaxed as possible.

If your knees want to bend during Stage 3, then allow them to do so. They will stay straighter with time, as your body becomes more flexible. Be patient!

Cross-Legged Sequence

This pose consists of a very versatile series of movements, stretching and strengthening the waist, lower back, hips and thighs. **Cross-Legged Sequence** *is particularly beneficial for anyone with a lower back problem, as the final stage of this pose realigns the lumbar vertebrae and surrounding muscles.*

Part 1:

- Sit in a loose cross-legged position, with the palms of your hands resting on your knees. Sit tall, with your shoulders drawn back and your tailbone pressed out to ensure that your back is straight. Your head should be upright. Take 3 deep breaths, aiming to sit taller, lengthening your spine a little more, with every breath out.

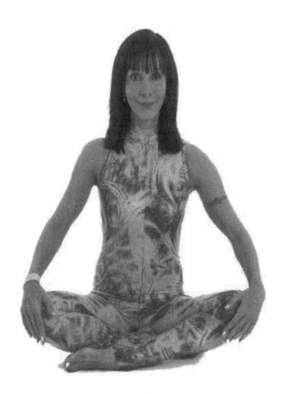

- Turn your body from your waist to face your right-hand side, placing your left hand on your right knee, and your right hand on the floor behind you, close to your bottom. Turn your head as though you were trying to look over your right shoulder. You are now in a seated spinal twist. Take 3 deep breaths, and return to your starting position with both hands over your knees.

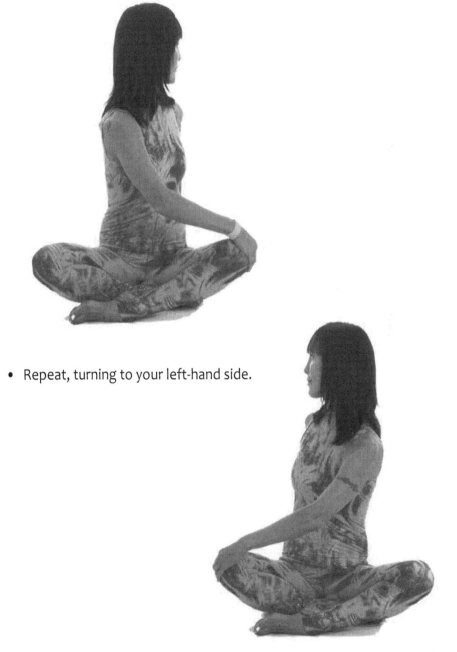

- Repeat, turning to your left-hand side.

Part 2:

- From the same starting position, place your left hand on the floor at your side, bend your elbow slightly and lean on your left arm. As you breathe in raise your right arm, and as you breathe out , stretch both your arm and your body over to your left-hand side. You should be aware of a stretch running down the right-hand side of your torso. When you feel ready, slowly increase your stretch by sliding your left hand further out to the side. Make sure you do not go so far that the right side of your bottom lifts off the floor. If this happens, slide your hand back in until your bottom returns to the floor. Hold this position for 3-5 deep breaths. Return to your starting position.

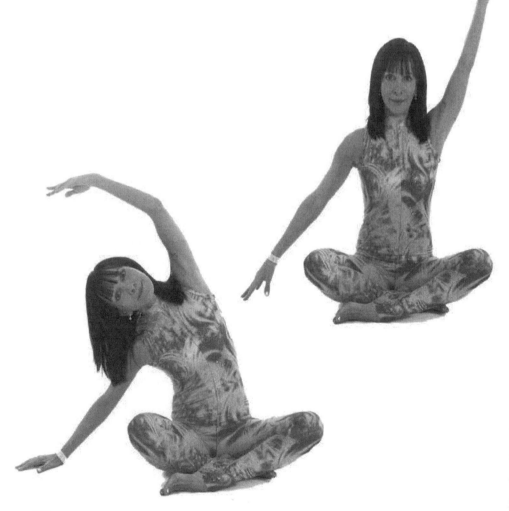

- Repeat with your left arm raised, stretching over to the right.

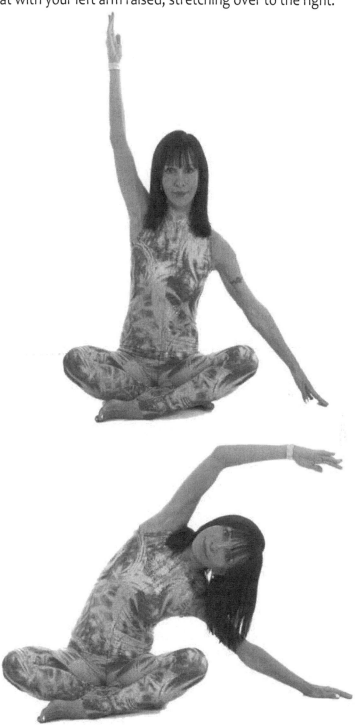

Part 3:

- From the same starting position, with both hands on your knees, take a deep breath in and as you breathe out draw your chest down towards the floor in front of you, allowing your hands to come off your knees and onto the floor in front of each knee. When you have dropped down as low as you can go, allow your head to relax and drop too – the weight of your head will increase the stretch a little. Stay here for 5 deep breaths, relaxing a little more with every breath out.

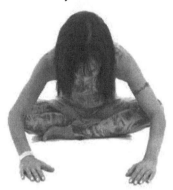

- If you are a little more flexible, you may be able to drop your elbows down onto the floor, and place your hands in **Prayer Pose**, for a stronger stretch.

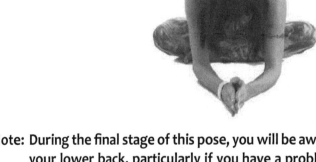

Note: During the final stage of this pose, you will be aware of a deep stretch in your lower back, particularly if you have a problem in this area. Often, with lower back problems, the muscles around the problem area can go into spasm, causing them to pull on the lumbar vertebrae, which in turn become misaligned. This lumbar spine realigning stretch can help to bring both vertebrae and surrounding muscles back into line, and can be extremely beneficial. Try to relax – remember to use your breath out to release any tension you may be feeling.

Seated Spinal Twist

By introducing a gentle rotation into the spine, **Seated Spinal Twist** *will keep your spine flexible and mobile. This pose also stretches your thighs and hips, easing out stiffness from the hip joints.*

- Sit with your knees bent, legs together, and feet on the floor.

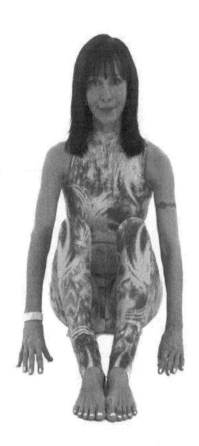

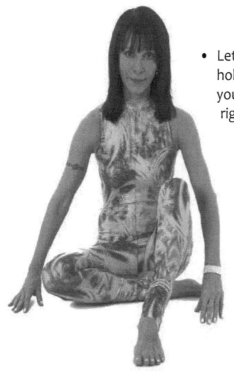

- Let your left knee drop out to the side. Take hold of your left ankle and draw it towards you, placing your left foot underneath your right thigh.

- Lift your right foot, and take it across your left leg, placing it on the floor to the outside of your thigh. (You can use your hand here if you wish, to lift your foot). Sitting upright, turn your body to the right and "hook" your left elbow over your right knee, drawing your knee gently towards your body with your arm. Place your right hand on the floor directly behind your bottom. Turn your head to the right, as though you are trying to look over your shoulder.

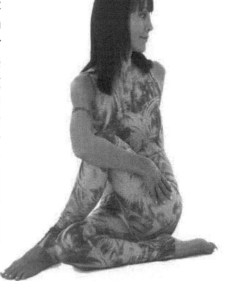

- Hold the pose for 5 deep breaths.

- Repeat each of the above stages to the other side.

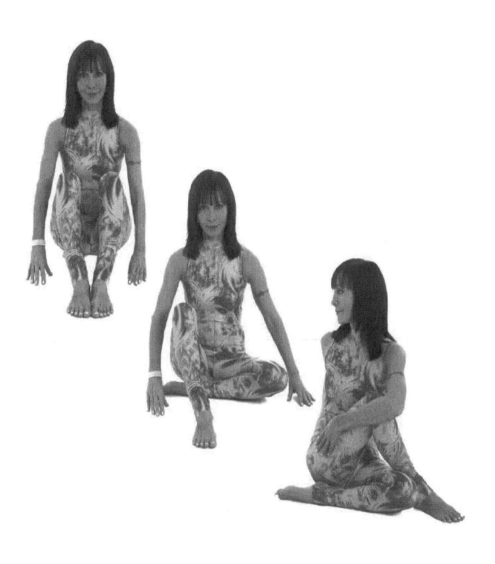

Note: If you cannot manage to "hook" your elbow over your knee, just use your hand instead. Try not to lean too heavily on your supporting arm, and keep this arm close to your body and as straight as possible, so that it acts like a "splint" to keep your spine straight and upright.

Kite Pose

Kite is a great flexibility pose which also gives the core stability muscles a strong workout. Remember, the stronger your core stability muscles, the less likely you are to have a problem with your back, hips or knees. Strong core stability muscles will also improve your posture and body alignment.

- Sit on the floor with your knees bent, and your feet on the floor in front of you. Relax and round your spine, and take hold of your insteps – your arms should be straight, and to the inside of your legs.

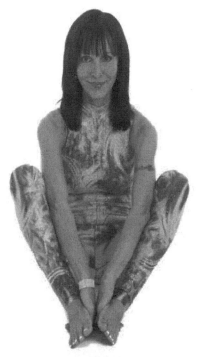

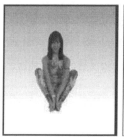 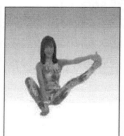 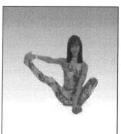 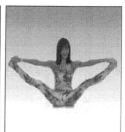

- Still holding both feet, slowly lift your right foot and stretch your leg out on a diagonal. Don't worry if you cannot get your leg straight – it can remain bent. Once you have brought your leg into this position, try to stretch and straighten your back, lengthening your neck, and sit as tall as you can. Hold for 2-3 deep breaths.

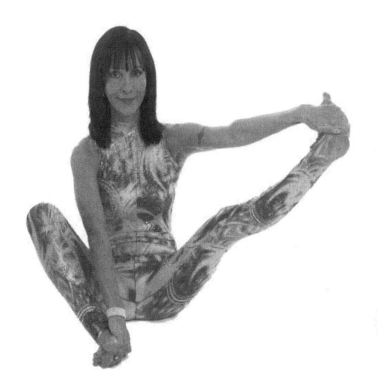

- Allow your back to relax, bend your right knee and return your foot to the floor.

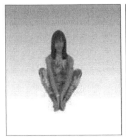 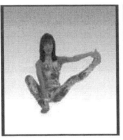 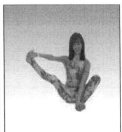 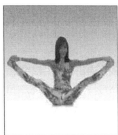

- Repeat with your left leg.

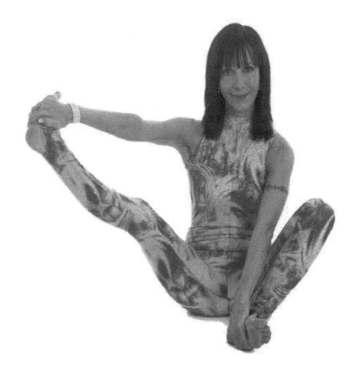

- Allow your back to relax, bend your left knee and return your foot to the floor.

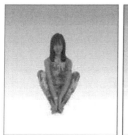 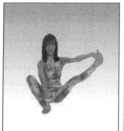 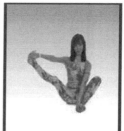 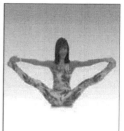

- Still holding both insteps, "walk" your feet in a few inches, which will bring you more onto your bottom, until you reach a point where you can lift both feet just an inch off the floor and keep balanced. Slowly, start to extend each leg out onto a diagonal – you can try this one leg at a time, or both legs at the same time. When you have straightened out your legs as far as you can comfortably manage, try to straighten your spine, sitting a little taller, extending your neck and drawing your shoulders back.

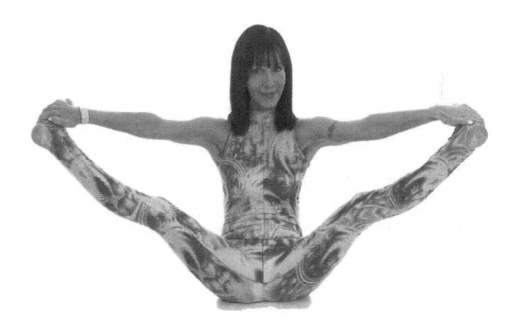

- You are now in **Kite Pose**! Try to hold the pose for 5 deep breaths, before bending your knees and returning your feet to the floor.

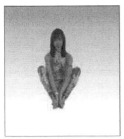 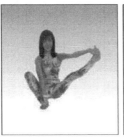 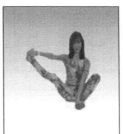 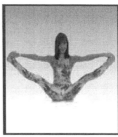

- Over time, once you have mastered *Kite Pose*, you might want to attempt a more advanced version by releasing your legs, and bringing your arms into an extended *Prayer Pose* inside your legs. An "optional extra" for you to work towards!

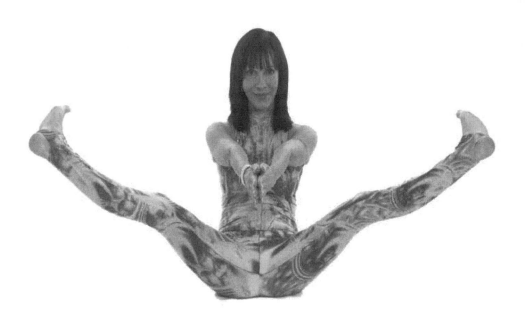

Note: In Kite Pose you will be aware of your core stability muscles working – that little tremor in the abdominal area – as well as the stretch in your legs, spine and shoulders. If you have difficulty in balancing, try to focus on something still in front of you, to help stabilise you.

During the final stage of Kite Pose, it is not uncommon to lose your balance and roll back to the floor! This is not a problem – but do make sure that you have a clear space behind you, for your safety.

Latch Pose

Latch Pose is a sequence of deep stretches for the thigh and pelvic area, which will both lengthen and strengthen the thigh muscles, and bring flexibility into the pelvis. A more flexible pelvis can improve your posture and reduce pressure and stress on the lumbar spine. Latch Pose is performed in two stages.

Stage 1:

- Come onto your hands and knees – your hands should be placed directly underneath your shoulders and your knees underneath your hips. Make sure your knees are well protected and comfortable.

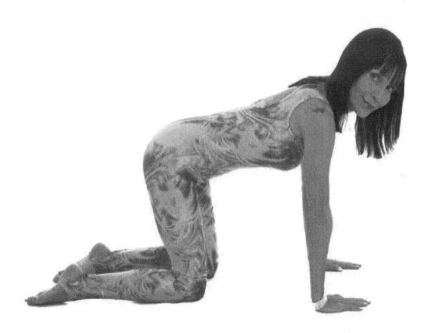

- Step your left foot forward, and place it on the floor just ahead of shoulder level.

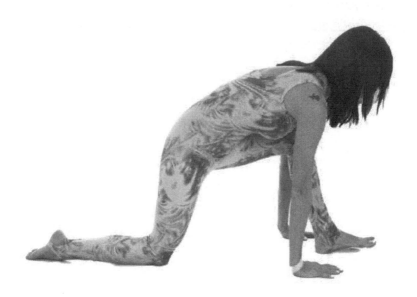

- Lift your torso into an upright position, and bring your hands into **Prayer Pose.**

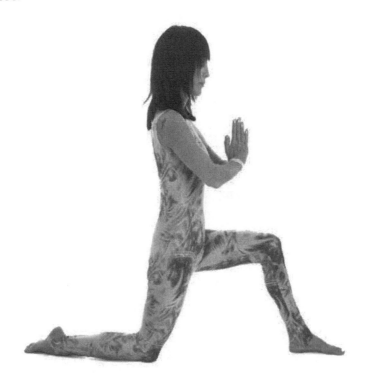

- Lunge deeply and slowly by pressing your hips forward – drawing your right thigh down towards the floor. Your bodyweight should be mainly on your left leg, and your left foot should remain completely on the floor with your heel directly underneath your knee. (Correct your foot position if necessary). You should feel a strong stretch in your right thigh. Keep your body upright, your shoulders back and your neck in line with your spine. Hold this stretch for 3-5 deep breaths.

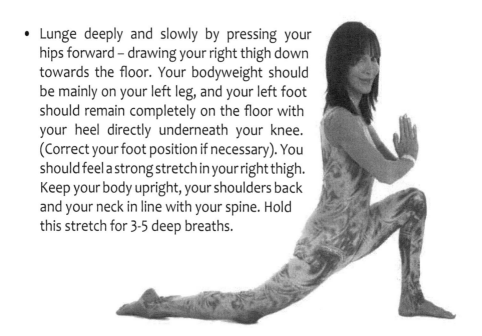

- Return your hands to the floor, and step your left foot back into your starting position.

- Repeat the above steps with your other leg.

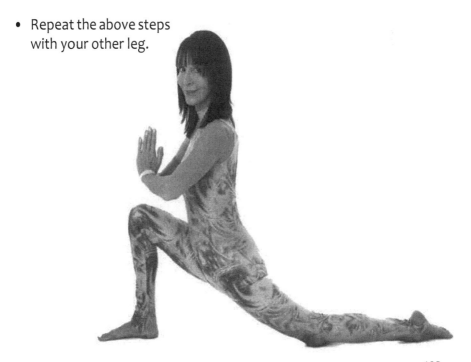

Stage 2:

- Come high onto your knees, with your body upright and arms by your sides.

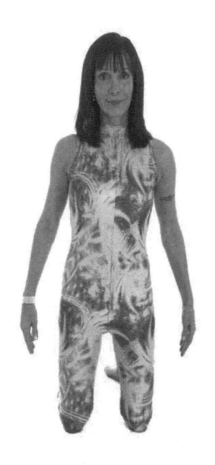

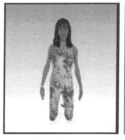 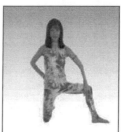 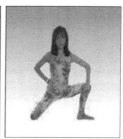

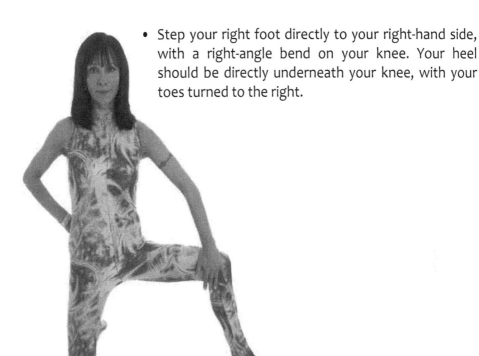

- Step your right foot directly to your right-hand side, with a right-angle bend on your knee. Your heel should be directly underneath your knee, with your toes turned to the right.

- Place the palm of your right hand to the inside of your right knee, and the palm of your left hand to the small of your back. Your right hand should be used to gently keep your knee in place and stop it from turning inwards, and your left hand should be used to ensure that your lower back does not arch. If you feel it arching, correct this with a pelvic tilt. Now slowly lunge sideways to your right – using both hands as described above – until you feel a strong stretch on both inner thighs.

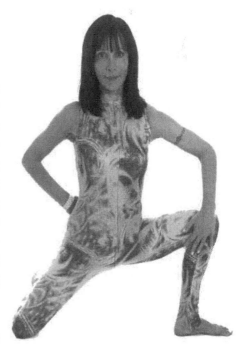

- Hold this stretch for 3-5 deep breaths.

- Return to your starting position.

- Repeat the above steps with your left leg.

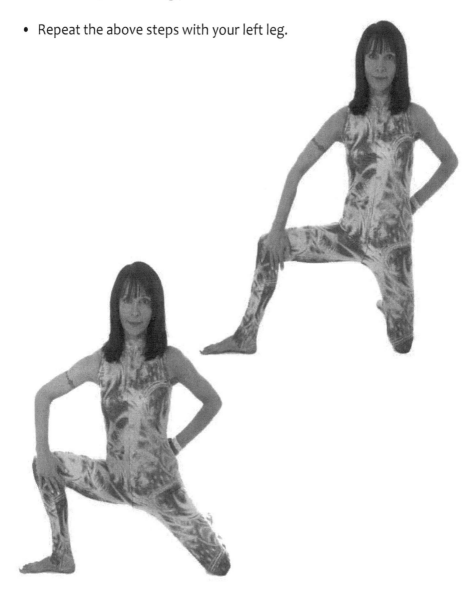

Note: Latch Pose consists of deep stretches which should be executed slowly and with care. Take your time and stretch gently – as your body becomes more flexible your stretches will naturally deepen. This process must not be rushed.

Make sure you have adequate padding under your knees during Latch Pose.

Lizard Pose

Lizard Pose is an intense pelvic, hip and thigh stretch. This is a wonderful stretch for those who want to increase their flexibility, and while it is a strong stretch, it is performed in 2 stages and you can stop after the first stage, building up to the final stage of the pose in your own time.

Lizard is performed from **Incline Plank Pose.**

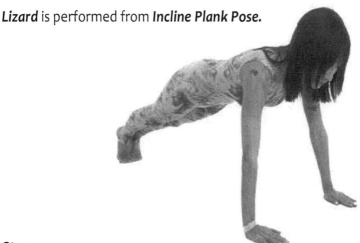

Stage 1:

- From **Incline Plank,** Step your right foot forwards, aiming to get the heel of your foot level with the heel of your right hand – your foot should be placed to the outside of your hand. If your foot did not come far enough forwards, take hold of your ankle and manually bring it into line. Press your right knee into your body – do not allow it to splay out.

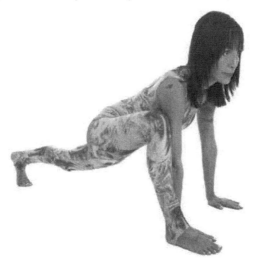

- You will feel the stretch immediately, in the pelvic area and also running down the front of your left thigh. Hold this stage of the pose for 3-5 deep breaths, gently easing your hips downwards.

- If this feels a deep enough stretch for you, finish the pose at this stage by stepping back with your right foot, returning to **Incline Plank**, and repeat **Stage 1** with your left leg.

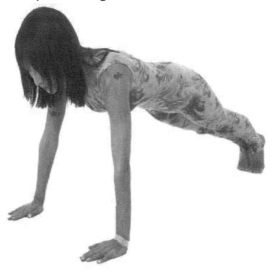

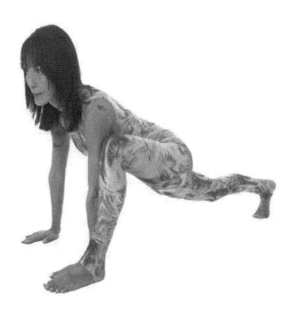

Stage 2:

- To complete **Lizard Pose,** drop down gently onto your left elbow. This will increase the stretch in your pelvic and thigh area considerably. Follow this with your right elbow when you are ready. When you are able to get both elbows down onto the floor, fold your arms one on top of the other. Your right knee should remain close to your side.

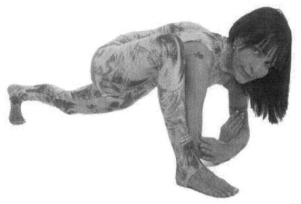

- You are now in full **Lizard Pose.** Hold for a further 3-5 deep breaths, and then push back on to your hands and step your right foot back, returning to **Incline Plank.**

- Repeat **Stage 2** with your left leg.

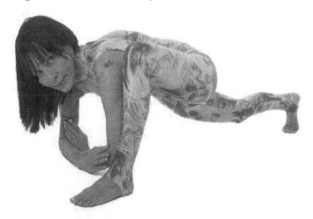

Note: Do not move on to the second – and final - stage of the pose until you feel you are suitably flexible enough. You should be able to complete the first stage of the pose, described above, comfortably before you progress to the final stage.

Praying Mantis Pose

Praying Mantis is a spectacular looking pose, providing a deep shoulder and neck stretch. It will ease stiff necks and loosen up the shoulders, increasing mobility in both areas. The pose is performed in two stages - the second stage of this pose also activates and strengthens the core stability muscles.

Stage 1:

- Come onto your hands and knees – your hands should be placed directly underneath your shoulders and your knees underneath your hips.

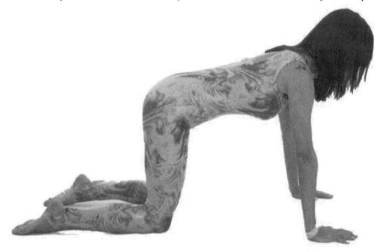

- Lift your right hand and pass your arm through the space between your left arm and leg. Allow your left elbow to bend, and come to rest your right shoulder and your head on the floor.

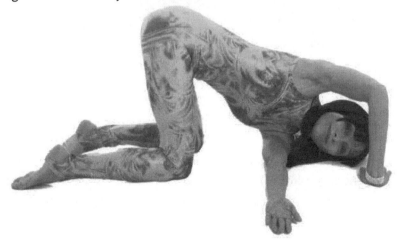

- Gently push against the floor with your left hand, to bring as much of your right shoulder onto the floor as possible.

- Tuck the toes of your left foot, and without lifting it off the floor slide it out until your leg is straight.

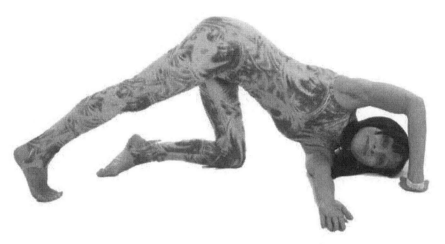

- Come into a high **Prayer Pose** with your hands – to do this, bend your right elbow and lift the palm of your right hand so it faces the ceiling. Place your left hand on top of your right hand, with your left elbow pointed to the ceiling.

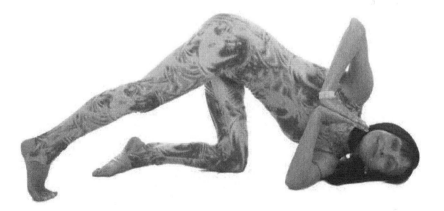

- You are now in the first stage of **Praying Mantis Pose**. Hold for 5 deep breaths.

Stage 2:

- Release your **Prayer Pose,** and return your left hand to the floor for support. Your right arm can simply relax again on the floor.

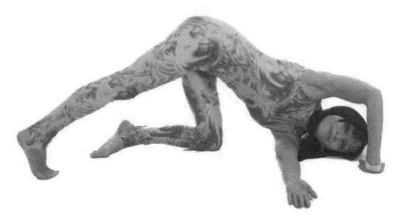

- Very slowly, start to raise your left leg, keeping it straight and toes pointed, as high towards the ceiling as you can. You should immediately feel the tell-tale sign of the activation of your core stability muscles – a slight tremor in the core area of your body.

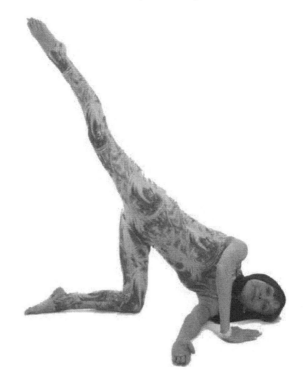

- When you feel ready, once again return your arms into a high **Prayer Pose** which will work your core stability muscles even harder. This is entirely optional – you can choose to continue supporting your pose by keeping your left hand on the floor.

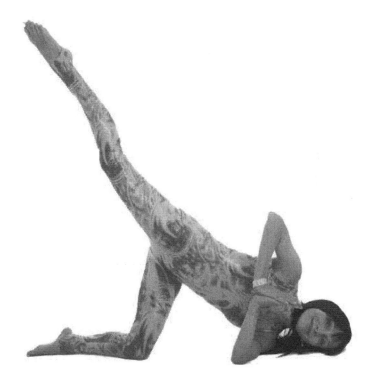

- Hold for 3 deep breaths and then bend your knee and replace it on the floor. Use your left hand to push yourself back onto your hands and knees.

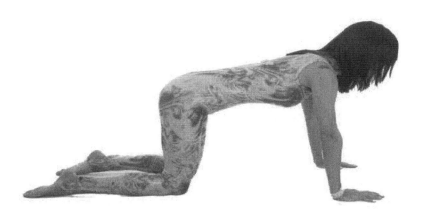

- Repeat both stages of the pose to the other side, extending and raising your right leg.

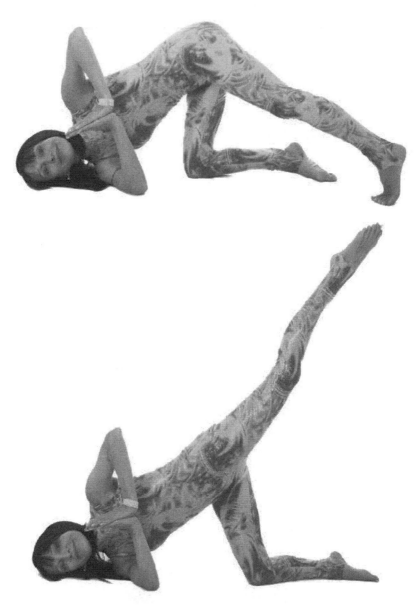

Note: Though tempting, do not tuck the toes of your supporting foot. If you do, you are allowing your foot to stabilise your position instead of your core stability muscles. Take your time with this pose ... become comfortable with Stage 1 first, before progressing to Stage 2.

Pigeon Pose

Pigeon Pose is amazing! *It is a weight bearing pose, and can help to improve bone density of the hips. Osteoporosis (brittle bones) will affect 1 woman in 3, and the hip is one of the most common areas of the body to suffer loss of bone density. If you already have a bone density problem in the hip, this pose can actually help replenish and re-grow new bone so you can in fact improve your condition. In this pose, by creating a very strong stretch which culminates in the hip, we are able to fool the body into thinking we are putting stress on the hip joint, and bone-building cells, known as osteoblasts and osteocytes, are produced in the area of the stretch to protect the hip joint. This fantastic pose can go a long way to ensuring your hips stay healthy and strong. It is also a great toning stretch for the thighs.*

- Come onto your hands and knees.

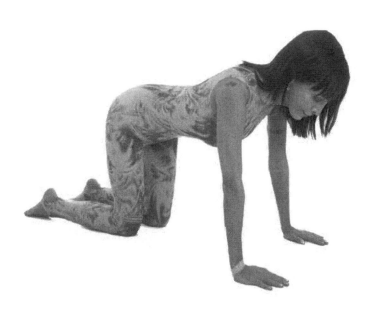

- Slide your left knee forwards, until it is between your hands, and also bring your left foot forwards (towards your right wrist). Sit down on the left side of your bottom. Make sure your bottom is actually in contact with the floor on that side. Try to straighten your right leg behind you, and turn your right knee down towards the floor as much as you can.

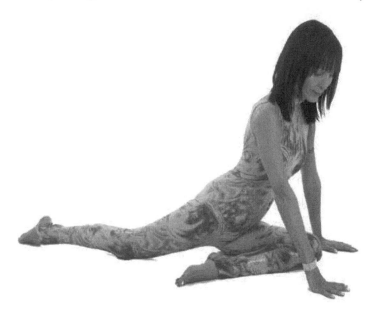

- Centre your body over your left knee, with your hands on the floor either side of your knee. Breathe in, and as you breathe out slowly walk your hands away, letting your body come down to rest on your left thigh. Rest your head and arms comfortably on the floor.

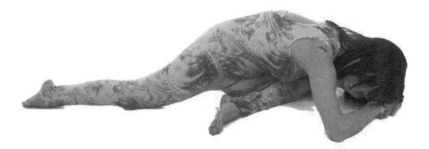

- You are now in **Pigeon Pose**. You should be aware of a deep stretch to the outside of your left thigh, radiating up to your hip. Your bodyweight resting on the thigh will intensify the stretch. Stay relaxed and hold the pose for 10-15 deep breaths.

- When you are ready to release your pose, slowly walk your hands back in, and when they are once again at shoulder level, use your arms to push yourself back onto hands and knees.

- Repeat with your other leg.

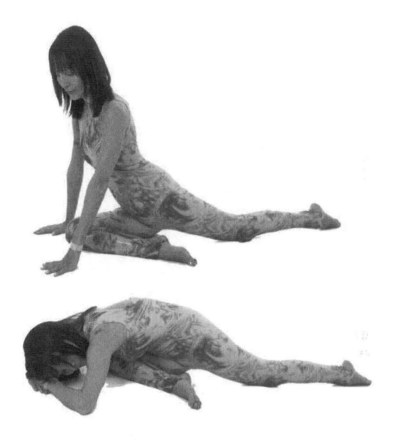

Note: It is important to relax completely in Pigeon Pose. This is harder than it sounds, as the resulting stretch is so deep it may make you involuntarily tense the muscles in your thigh. Be aware of this, and use your deep breathing to relax into the pose. Visualise the tension leaving your body with your breath out until you feel completely relaxed in the stretch. The more you can relax, the deeper – and more effective – the stretch becomes.

Loss of bone density does also affect men – approximately 1 in 12 men will be affected. However, it is largely hormone related which is why the figure is higher for women.

Wolf Seat

*Wolf Seat is another weight-bearing stretch for the hips, with exactly the same benefits as **Pigeon Pose** with regard to improving bone density of the hip. However, it is a stronger stretch for the hips and thighs, and should not be attempted until **Pigeon Pose** can be performed comfortably.*

- Come onto hands and knees.

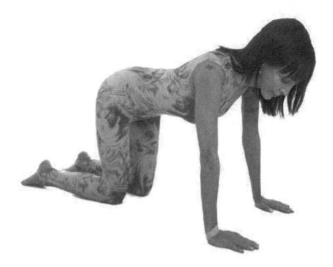

- Cross your right knee **behind** your left, making sure that your knee returns to the floor on the other side. Open your feet as wide as possible, into a "fishtail".

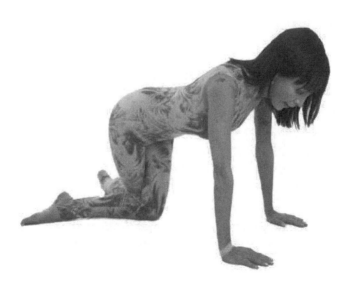

- Slowly, walk your hands in towards you and carefully lower your bottom down to sit on the floor in between your feet. You will be resting mainly on the right side of your bottom – the left side will be slightly raised. The aim is to have one knee directly on top of the other, with both legs stacked neatly in a V shape.

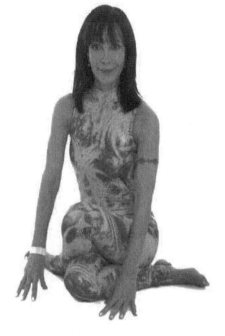

- To complete your pose, walk your hands away to bring your body forwards, over your legs. Keep your bodyweight supported on your arms. You will now feel the stretch increase considerably.

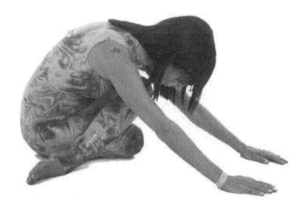

- Hold the pose for 5-10 deep breaths.

- When you are ready to come out of the pose, walk your hands back in, use your arms to push yourself back onto hands and knees, and uncross your legs.

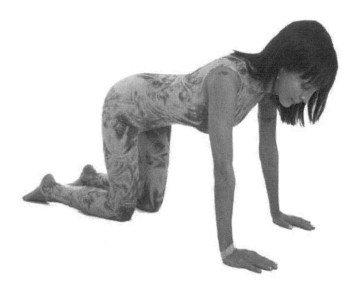

- Repeat the pose with your left knee crossed behind your right.

Note: In Wolf Seat you will immediately feel a very strong stretch in your thighs, radiating up towards your hips, and this stretch will feel more intense in the upper thigh. Stay as relaxed as possible to allow the stretch to develop and build up to its fullest level. Focus on your deep, slow breathing to relax, and visualise the tension melting away with every breath out.

Hamstring Vinyasa

Hamstrings are a group of muscles and tendons at the back of the thigh and knee. They are notorious for being tight and short, which makes them extremely vulnerable and easily damaged. Moreover, tight hamstrings are known to "tug" on the lower back muscles, and can even pull them out of alignment. They should be stretched regularly. This is a two-stage pose, incorporating both stretching and movement.

Part 1:

- Lie on your back, with your knees bent.

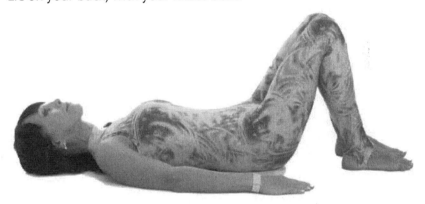

- Raise your left leg up towards the ceiling, toes pointed. Allow your knee to slightly bend, reach up and take hold around your calf muscle with both hands – the higher up towards your ankle you can hold, the better, but do not lift your head.

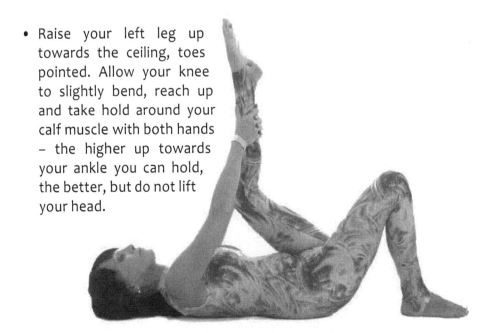

- Allow your knee to bend a little more, which should enable you to bring your thigh a little closer to your body. Now, try to straighten your leg – just a small amount, don't "lock" your leg straight. You should immediately feel the stretch behind your thigh. Stay as relaxed as you can, and breathe deeply. Hold this position for 3 deep breaths.

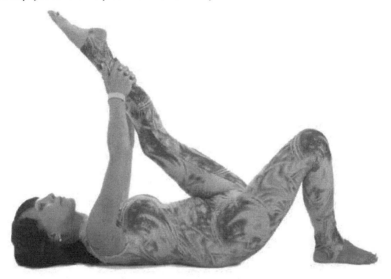

- Repeat this process again – another small bend on your knee, bring your thigh a little lower, and then straighten out your leg slightly.

- Repeat the above steps a third (and final) time, but this time, when you have straightened out your leg as far as you can comfortably manage, flex your foot – heel pressed up and toes pointing down - which will increase the stretch, bringing it into your calf as well.

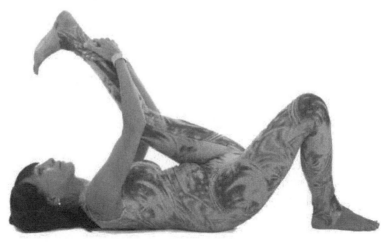

Part 2: (linking movements known as vinyasa)

- Still holding your leg as close to your body as you can comfortably manage, and with your foot still flexed, take a deep breath in and as you breathe out lift your upper body off the floor, bringing your chest towards your thigh.

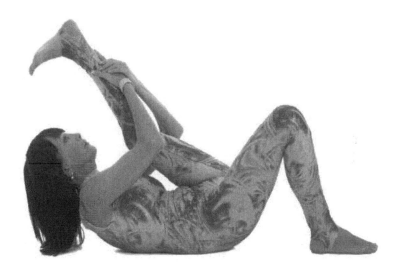

- Breathe in again, and as you breathe out this time slide your right foot out until your leg is straight and resting on the floor. At this stage your stretch is stronger, as you have added the weight of your body to the stretch, and extending your right leg increases the stretch even more. Hold this position if you can, for 2-3 deep breaths.

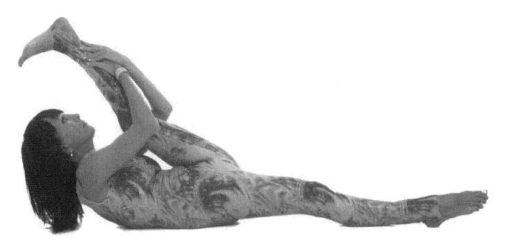

- Breathe in, and as you breathe out bend your right knee and slide your foot back into its original position.

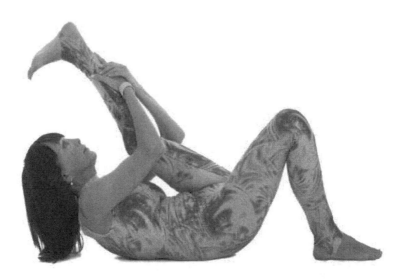

- Finally, breathe in and as you breathe out release your body to the floor and relax your left leg by bending your knee and return your foot to the floor.

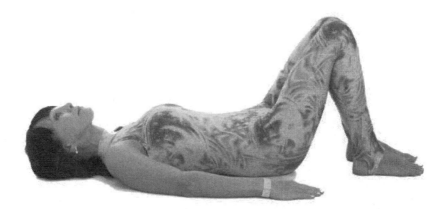

- Roll your head gently from side to side once or twice to release any tension that may have built up in your neck.

- Repeat from the beginning with your right leg raised.

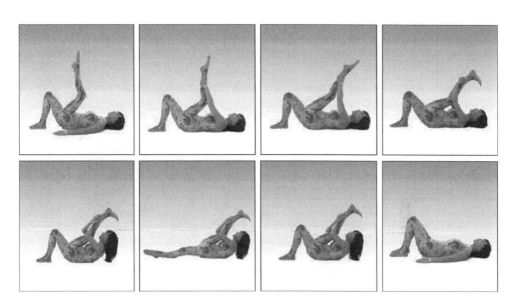

Note: After completing the first part of Hamstring Vinyasa, you will have brought your leg considerably closer to your body, thereby increasing the depth of your stretch. By doing this slowly, and in small increments – just an inch or two at a time - you are safely and effectively allowing the stretch to develop and your muscles to lengthen. This form of stretching is particularly effective, as the muscles will remain stretched for a longer period of time.

During the second part of the pose you add the weight of your body to the stretch which increases it even further. You will feel this.

Always take your time with your stretching, never rush it, and use your deep breathing to stay as relaxed as possible.

Downward Facing Dog Pose ("Downward Dog")

This inverted pose stretches the shoulders, pectoral muscles, spine and legs – particularly the hamstrings and calves. It also sends a good supply of oxygenated blood to the brain, making you feel refreshed and alert.

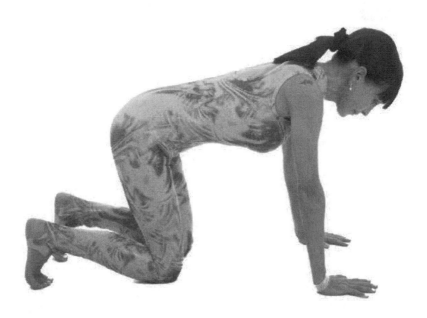

- Come onto hands and knees to start **Downward Dog.** Your hands should be slightly wider than shoulder width, and your knees should be together and directly under your hips. Tuck your toes.

- Take a deep breath in and as you breathe out straighten your legs, lifting your bottom up towards the ceiling. Keep your hands where they are – they should stay above head and shoulder level – and push against the floor, to bring the backs of your arms as close to the floor as possible. Press your tailbone high towards the ceiling. Your aim is to come into a sharp inverted "V" shape.

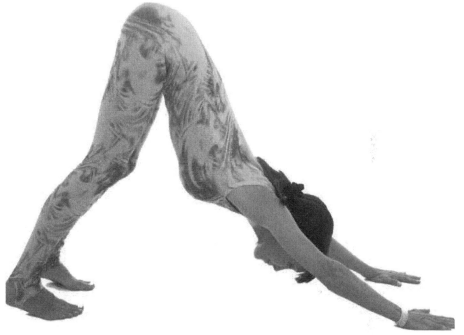

- Hold the pose for 5-8 deep breaths – continually pushing the backs of your arms toward the floor and your tailbone higher toward the ceiling each time you breathe out.

- To come out of **Downward Dog** safely, lift up onto your toes, bend your knees and lower them carefully to your mat. Drop into **Child Pose**, relax here for a few breaths, and uncurl slowly.

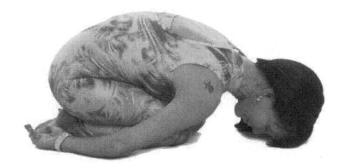

- Over time, when you are comfortable with your practice of **Downward Dog,** you might wish to consider taking it further by lifting your legs, one at a time, up towards the ceiling. This is a wonderful stretch! Don't worry if you cannot straighten your leg or lift it very high at first – this will get better as you become more flexible. Practice makes perfect!

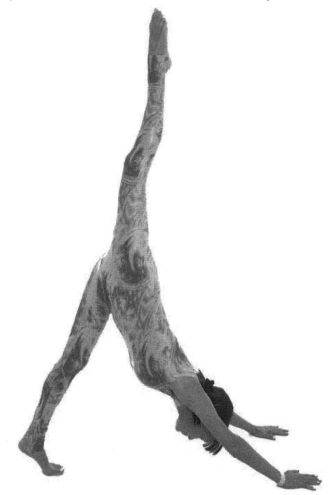

Note: In Downward Dog your legs do not need to be straight – slightly bent knees are fine – and your heels do not need to be on the floor, although you should try to keep them as close to the floor as you can manage.

During any inversion pose (where your head is in a dropped position like this) it is very important that you do not try to spring back to standing upright too quickly. This can cause your blood pressure to drop, and make you feel dizzy.

Carpal Stretch

*Carpal Stretch is a stress-relieving stretch for the wrists – particularly important if you have a job that requires a repetitive movement, increasing the risk of Repetitive Strain Injury (RSI). This simple stretch will minimise the risk of RSI, and Carpal Tunnel Syndrome – pressure on the Median nerve, as it passes through the wrist. A lot of Hatha Yoga poses require us to be on hands and knees, which can put pressure on the wrists, so I always think it's a good idea to practice **Carpal Stretch** at the end of your yoga routine.*

- Kneel on the floor, and sit your bottom on your heels. Stretch your arms straight out in front of you, and place your fingertips on the floor about 10-12" away from your knees, with your palms facing outward. Your arms should be straight.

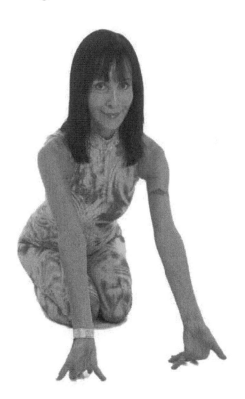

- Start to gently ease the palms of your hands downward towards the floor – without putting any weight on your arms. You should remain sitting on your heels.

- Stop as soon as you feel a very gentle stretch – from the inside of your wrists and up towards your elbows. When you feel the stretch, hold the pose still for 3-5 deep breaths.

- Now lift your hands and turn them over, so that the backs of your hands are facing outward and fingertips on the floor. Repeat the stretch – this time easing the backs of your hands toward the floor. Aim to go just beyond knuckle level, which should result in a gentle stretch running from the front of your wrists and up towards your elbows. Again, hold the stretch for 3 deep breaths.

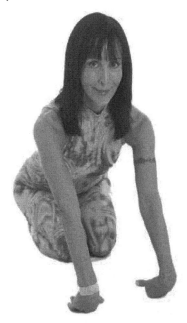

- To complete the pose, simply shake your hands gently several times.

Note: **You are not supposed to place the palms or the backs of your hands flat on the floor – just ease them down until you feel the stretch. If your hands easily go flat to the floor, take them further away from you. NEVER place your bodyweight on your arms in this position.**

If you cannot sit comfortably on your heels, sit with your legs stretched out in front of you, with your hands on the floor by your sides. Walk your hands as far away from you as you can, and then follow the above steps for Carpal Stretch.

For anyone at risk of RSI, practice this pose on a daily basis.

SECTION 7

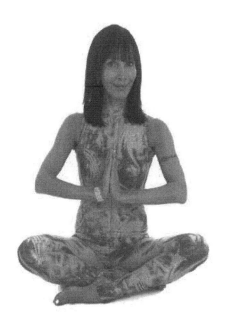

RELAXATION POSES

RELAXATION POSES

Relaxation poses do exactly that; they will enable you to slow your breathing down and relax every muscle of your body, and they can be used in between the more strenuous poses to simply release tension, rest and prepare for the next pose.

It is also recommended that a relaxation pose be used at the end of your yoga session as a cool-down. While in a relaxation pose, your heart rate and blood pressure will return to normal, leaving you prepared – both mentally and physically – for your next yoga pose, or to simply continue with your day.

Life can be stressful for us all, and it is well documented that stress can kill. We are living our lives at such a fast and frenzied pace, constantly under pressure, and to a large degree we have forgotten how to completely relax.

Starting today, try to take at least five minutes every day to learn the fine art of relaxation!

Corpse Pose

Corpse is not the most pleasant of names, but quite apt! **Corpse**, *paradoxically, is one of the most important, yet one of the physically least challenging, poses in Yoga! It is important because, with regular practice, it will teach you how to totally relax your mind, as well as every muscle, allowing the tension and stress you are holding inside to just dissolve away. Not as easy as it might sound!*

In **Corpse Pose** *your eyes should be closed – so you will need to read through the following steps first before you try it!*

- First, make sure you are warm and in a quiet room. If possible, dim or turn off the lights, or draw the curtains. You should not be wearing any restrictive clothing. Lie on your back on a yoga mat, on the floor. Make yourself comfortable, and close your eyes. Roll your head from side to side several times, before letting it come to rest in a comfortable central position, face towards the ceiling. Allow your feet to drift apart, arms resting down by your sides, palms of your hands facing up. Let your fingers curl and relax. Try to empty your mind of as many of your thoughts as you can, and focus instead on just your breathing. Start to slow each breath down, breathing more and more deeply. Each time you breathe in, feel the rise in your chest as you fill your body with air. And each time you breathe out, feel how your chest draws down as the air leaves your body. Start to make every breath a little slower, and a little deeper, than the one before.

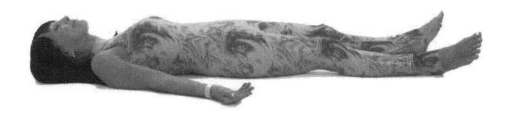

- As your breathing slows down, your body begins to relax more deeply. Tension is released from the muscles and leaves your body with your breath out. So . . . . with every breath out . . . . you are becoming more and more relaxed.

- Imagine yourself to be totally weightless, floating, empty your mind and relax.

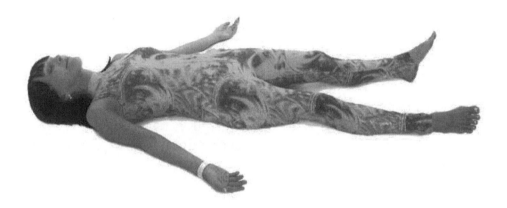

- Try to stay here, totally relaxed, and at peace with yourself, for at least five minutes. (An alarm clock might be a good idea – to stop you drifting off to sleep!) When you are ready to come out of the pose, focus on your breathing once more, allowing your mind to slowly acclimatise to your surroundings. Start to move your fingers, wriggle your toes, bringing life back into your hands and your feet.

- When you feel ready, open your eyes and bend your knees, placing your feet flat on the floor. To sit yourself up, hug your knees to your chest and start to rock gently back and forth, using a little momentum until, after several rocks, you stay seated.

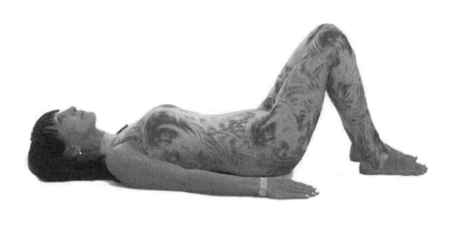

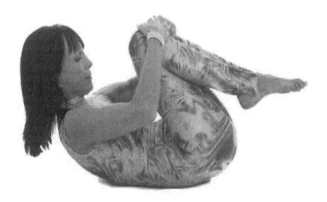

Note: Try to practice Corpse Pose on a daily basis for five minutes. You will soon start to feel all the benefits a relaxed mind and body can bring! Corpse can be done as an isolated pose – whenever you feel the need to relax – but I also recommend that your yoga practice should always be completed with this pose.

Child Pose

*This is a wonderful relaxation pose for spine, shoulders and neck. You will find that I suggest you come into **Child Pose** after certain poses in this book, as a way of relaxing the body and refreshing the mind.*

- From hands and knees, drop your bottom down to rest on your heels, and your chest to your thighs. Your forehead should rest on the floor – but if it does not reach, place a cushion on the floor in front of you for your head to rest on.

- Bring your arms down by your sides, so that your hands are level with your feet. Relax your shoulders and let them "drop" down towards the floor.

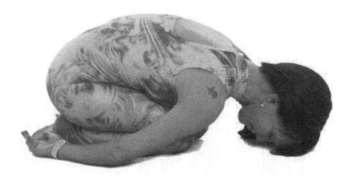

- You are now in **Child Pose.** Stay in this pose for up to one minute, breathing slowly and deeply, before uncurling, vertebra by vertebra, with your head coming up last.

Extended Arm Child Pose

*This is simply a variation on the standard **Child Pose** – another great stretch for the spine and shoulders.*

- From hands and knees, drop your bottom down to rest on your heels, and your chest to your thighs. Your forehead should rest on the floor – but if it does not reach, place a cushion on the floor in front of you for your head to rest on.

- Stretch your arms out in front of you, with the palms of your hands resting on the floor.

- Walk your fingertips away as far as possible, and then gently ease your elbows closer to the floor to bring on a deeper shoulder stretch.

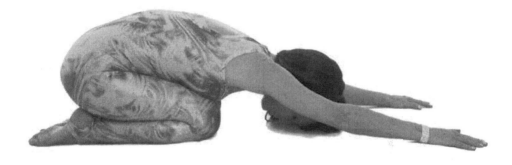

- Stay in this position, with your arms extended, for approximately one minute. You may then uncurl slowly, or link this pose with **Child Pose** by bringing your arms straight down by your sides, shoulders dropped, and relax here for a further minute.

Note: If you are quite flexible, you can increase the depth of the stretch in Extended Arm Child Pose by taking your knees and thighs out wider, enabling your body to drop closer to the floor in between your thighs.

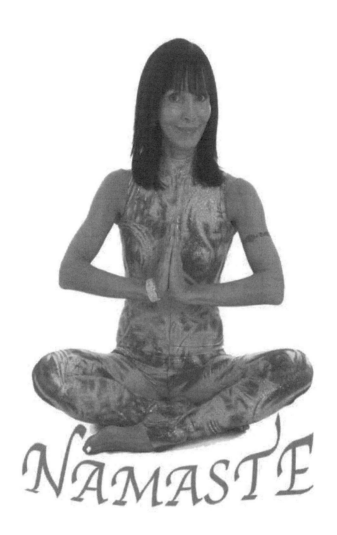